T0296673

CHRONIC FAILURES

MEDICAL ANTHROPOLOGY:
HEALTH, INEQUALITY, AND SOCIAL JUSTICE
Series editor: Lenore Manderson

Books in the Medical Anthropology series are concerned with social patterns of and social responses to ill health, disease, and suffering, and how social exclusion and social justice shape health and healing outcomes. The series is designed to reflect the diversity of contemporary medical anthropological research and writing, and will offer scholars a forum to publish work that showcases the theoretical sophistication, methodological soundness, and ethnographic richness of the field.

Books in the series may include studies on the organization and movement of peoples, technologies, and treatments, how inequalities pattern access to these, and how individuals, communities and states respond to various assaults on wellbeing, including from illness, disaster, and violence.

Ellen Block and Will McGrath, *Infected Kin: Orphan Care and AIDS in Lesotho*
Jessica Hardin, *Faith and the Pursuit of Health: Cardiometabolic Disorders in Samoa*
Carina Heckert, *Fault Lines of Care: Gender, HIV, and Global Health in Bolivia*
Alison Heller, *Fistula Politics: Birthing Injuries and the Quest for Continence in Niger*
Ciara Kierans, *Chronic Failures: Kidneys, Regimes of Care, and the Mexican State*
Nolan Kline, *Pathogenic Policing: Immigration Enforcement and Health in the U.S. South*
Joel Christian Reed, *Landscapes of Activism: Civil Society and HIV and AIDS Care in Northern Mozambique*
Beatriz M. Reyes-Foster, *Psychiatric Encounters: Madness and Modernity in Yucatan, Mexico*
Sonja van Wichelen, *Legitimating Life: Adoption in the Age of Globalization and Biotechnology*
Lesley Jo Weaver, *Sugar and Tension: Diabetes and Gender in Modern India*
Andrea Whittaker, *International Surrogacy as Disruptive Industry in Southeast Asia*

CHRONIC FAILURES

Kidneys, Regimes of Care, and the Mexican State

CIARA KIERANS

RUTGERS UNIVERSITY PRESS

New Brunswick, Camden, and Newark, New Jersey, and London

Library of Congress Cataloging-in-Publication Data
Names: Kierans, Ciara, author.
Title: Chronic failures: kidneys, regimes of care, and the Mexican state /
    Ciara Kierans.
Description: New Brunswick: Rutgers University Press, 2019. | Series: Medical
    anthropology: health, inequality, and social justice | Includes bibliographical
    references and index.
Identifiers: LCCN 2019006135 | ISBN 9780813596655 (cloth) |
    ISBN 9780813596648 (pbk.)
Subjects: | MESH: Kidney Failure, Chronic—therapy | Kidney Failure,
    Chronic—ethnology | Healthcare Disparities | Kidney Transplantation—
    economics | Health Services Accessibility | Socioeconomic Factors | Mexico
Classification: LCC RC918.R4 | NLM WJ 342 | DDC 616.6/14—dc23
LC record available at https://lccn.loc.gov/2019006135

A British Cataloging-in-Publication record for this book is available from the
British Library.

All photographs by the author

♾ The paper used in this publication meets the requirements of the American National
Standard for Information Sciences—Permanence of Paper for Printed Library
Materials, ANSI Z39.48-1992.

www.rutgersuniversitypress.org

Manufactured in the United States of America

For my loving parents,
my mother, Molly, and in memory of my father, Tommy

CONTENTS

FOREWORD

LENORE MANDERSON

Medical Anthropology: Health, Inequality, and Social Justice is a new series from Rutgers University Press, designed to capture the diversity of contemporary medical anthropological research and writing. The beauty of ethnography is its capacity, through storytelling, to make sense of suffering as a social experience, and to set it in context. This series is concerned with health and illness, and inequality and social justice, and central to this are the ways that social structures and ideologies shape the likelihood and impact of infections, injuries, bodily ruptures and disease, chronic conditions and disability, treatment and care, and social repair and death.

The brief for this series is broad. The books are concerned with health and illness, healing practices, and access to care, but the authors illustrate too the importance of context—of geography, physical condition, service availability, and income. Health and illness are social facts; the circumstances of the maintenance and loss of health are always and everywhere shaped by structural, global, and local relations. Society, culture, economy, and political organization as much as ecology shape the variance of illness, disability, and disadvantage. But as medical anthropologists have long illustrated, the relationships between social context and health status are complex. In addressing these questions, the authors in this series showcase the theoretical sophistication, methodological rigor, and empirical richness of the field, while expanding a map of illness, and social and institutional life, to illustrate the effects of material conditions and social meanings in troubling and surprising ways.

The books in the series move across social circumstances, health conditions, and geography, as well as their intersections and interactions, to demonstrate how individuals, communities, and states manage assaults on wellbeing. The books reflect medical anthropology as a constantly changing field of scholarship, drawing diversely on research in residential and virtual communities, clinics, and laboratories; in emergency care and public health settings; with service providers, individual healers, and households; and with social bodies, human bodies, and biologies. Although medical anthropology once concentrated on systems of healing, particular diseases and embodied experiences, today, the field has expanded to include environmental disaster and war, science, technology and faith, gender-based violence, and forced migration. Curiosity about the body and its vicissitudes remains a pivot for our work, but our concerns are with the location of bodies in social life, and with how social structures, temporal imperatives, and shifting exigencies shape life courses. This dynamic field reflects an ethics of the discipline to address these pressing issues of our time.

Globalization has contributed to and adds to the complexity of influences on health outcomes; it (re)produces social and economic relations that institutionalize poverty, unequal conditions of everyday life and work, and environments in which diseases increase or subside. Globalization patterns the movement and relations of peoples, technologies and knowledge, and programs and treatments; it shapes differences in health experiences and outcomes across space; and it informs and amplifies inequalities at individual and country levels. Global forces and local inequalities compound and constantly load on individuals to impact their physical and mental health, and their households and communities. At the same time, as the subtitle of this series indicates, we are concerned with questions of social exclusion and inclusion, social justice, and repair—again both globally and in local settings. The books will challenge readers not only to reflect on sickness and suffering, deficit, and despair, but also on resistance and restitution—on how people respond to injustices and evade the fault lines that might seem to predetermine life outcomes. Although not all of the books take this direction, the aim is to widen the frame within which we conceptualize embodiment and suffering.

Nowhere are the fault lines that shape life outcomes as clear as in organ failure, dialysis, transplantation, and the high costs of subsequent life-long medication. In *Chronic Failures: Kidneys, Regimes of Care, and the Mexican State*, Ciara Kierans powerfully illustrates the uneven distributions of risk, illness, care, clinical treatment, and survival in the case of chronic kidney disease (CKD).

CKD can be the consequence of a congenital anomaly, but its most common causes are contextual, social, and economic. Diabetes and hypertension are the primary causes of chronic kidney disease (CKD) globally, and diabetes affects around one in eleven people worldwide. Mexico has the highest death rate in the world from CKD, and diabetes is its leading cause of death and disability, largely in association with overweight and obesity and driven by food insecurity, poverty, and the relative affordability and aggressive marketing of foods high in salt and sugar. But other factors drive CKD too. Infectious diseases as well as diabetes, from various bacteria, viruses, and autoimmune conditions, may all result in kidney damage; CKD of unknown etiology (CKDu), likely associated with soil and food contamination and so tied to the environment, conditions of labor, and poor infrastructure, is also especially prevalent in resource-poor communities. Those whose kidneys have failed need urgent and lifelong medical care. For poor families without health insurance, the direct and indirect costs of care can be debilitating and overwhelming.

Ciara Kierans's ethnography is set is Guadalajara, the capital city of Jalisco state—seven hours by car northwest of Mexico City, a relatively large city with sophisticated medical services and technologies that contrast with those in other more impoverished states. But here as elsewhere, CKD is highly prevalent, and the experiences of people in Guadalajara reflect nationwide experiences. Although effective strategies are available to delay disease progression and reduce deaths due directly or indirectly to CKD, inequality shapes how this plays out. Wealth and poverty determine who, how, and when a person has access to specialist nephrologists and nurses, who can chose home (peritoneal) dialysis or clinic-based hemodialysis, and what this choice might mean on an everyday basis to them and their kin. Personal relationships and willingness to donate, as well as blood and tissue compatibility, determine the feasibility of kidney donation, but household finances shape the possibility, timing, and conditions of the transplant. Social workers, charities, and money lenders need to be mobilized for personal support and financial aid to proceed, and to ensure subsequently the ongoing supply of autoimmune suppressant medication to prevent organ rejection. For those who experience transplant rejection or later failure, and have the opportunity for a new transplant, this is a repetitive process. As medical staff, clinics, equipment, organs, protocols, pharmaceuticals, and paper-work interplay, they expose the roles of networks and instruments of the state, the market, and society in exacerbating the inequalities of the disease complex.

Ciara Kierans's ethnography provides us with a compelling and sophisticated demonstration of assemblage, as a network of arrangements that takes its complexity from the uniqueness of the setting. The suffering, experiences, and sacrifices of patients and their families provide an affective entry point to renal disease and care, but more shocking—perhaps surprisingly—are the complicated interlockings of institutions, protocol, and professionals, and the administrative processes that shape their routine tasks. Much of the work that goes on under these banners—making appointments, matching an organ and prioritizing surgery, filling in forms, interpreting computer tomography—is mute or irrelevant to a patient with ready access to quality care. For the majority of people with CKD, however, everyday life and individual health is precarious; without insurance, they struggle to access the resources, affordances, and capital on which treatment and care is predicated. *Chronic Failures* provides a chilling account of the political economy, biopolitics, and bureaucracy of the transplants complex, and of the persistent, petty insults inherent in the health system that stand between patients and their possible survival.

PROLOGUE

This book is about regimes of renal care—that organizational constellation that makes up and generates transplant medicine—as it is encountered in Mexico by uninsured patients and their families. I approach these regimes in their locally fashioned and occasioned terms. I am interested in their politics and affordances: how these biotechnical interventions can be mobilized and made to work across different places, by different social actors, for different reasons, and with variable effects. My own encounters with transplant medicine, as an anthropologist, have taught me much about its multiplicities, about the capacity of this branch of medicine to extend itself beyond the clinic, to spill out into social, cultural, political, and economic domains, to be shaped by them and to shape them in turn.

This book, though ostensibly about Mexico, is an outcome of these encounters. More than twenty years ago, as an Irish doctoral student in anthropology, I tracked and traced the trajectories of Irish patients with chronic kidney disease (CKD)—dialysis patients and organ transplant recipients—in an attempt to generate an existential and culturally contextual account of their lives. I wanted to understand the world-making possibilities and everyday-life constraints bound up with transplant technologies and how receiving the so-called gift of the donated organ conferred on patients particular commitments and obligations. I wanted to know what stories could and could not be told about the respective successes and failures of the organ transplant in a context where stories and gifts have distinct cultural values. Among other things, what I learned was that my questions and concerns were not merely disciplinary; the questions and concerns of a fledgling anthropologist. They were first and foremost the questions of the patients I spoke with, travelled to dialysis with, and lived with after they received an organ transplant. They were also the questions and concerns of their family members and friends, as well as their doctors, nurses, psychologists, and all those charged with their care and support. I learned that ethnographic work, as Holmes and Marcus (2008) describe, is a work of alignment; the recognition that we are, all together, attempting to make sense of the same human terrain.

Moving to the UK, as an academic and research anthropologist, generated further opportunities to interrogate the workings of transplant medicine, albeit in a different social and cultural context. Unlike Ireland, which had been in the mid-1990s still a relatively homogeneous country—where issues of health, medicine, and the human body were not so culturally differentiated—within the UK, organ donation and allocation were cached out in other terms—those of race, ethnicity, and the inequalities they reflected. In this context, the sourcing and allocation of organs-for-transplant had been culturalized as a problem of and for members of the so-called minority ethnic communities who needed them most, but who donated them least. This problem invited another tracking and tracing—one I undertook with my colleague Jessie Cooper—back into the laboratories and clinical settings where those problems emerged, where organs are matched between various givers and receivers. This provided an opportunity to understand how scientific and technical concerns—algorithmic equations, laboratory practice, institutional contingencies, and organizational processes—are part of the deep social and cultural infrastructures of organ transfer. These settings revealed the mundane and routine work of the laboratory technicians and medical staff who must arbitrate between the giving and receiving of organs. Again, what emerged as intellectual problems for the anthropologist started first as practical problems for the social actors that inhabited this ethnographic terrain. Not only are our anthropological questions already in the world, others are equally invested in making sense of them; of resolving them. The ethnographic ground of sense-making is, thus, a shared one. Understanding this has shaped my approach to regimes of renal care and the technologies of transplantation in Mexico as a constellation of human practice, social need, political will, and expedience. Regimes of renal care are dependent on different medical, political, and institutional arrangements; different organ donation practices (predominantly living-related in Mexico as opposed to predominantly deceased in Ireland and the UK); a different political-economy of health, one which has placed access to transplant medicine outside (as opposed to inside) welfare arrangements for those most vulnerable to the condition of kidney disease and, therefore, profoundly expensive. The high cost of renal care carries resource implications for those who require, as well as those who provide, perform, and administer, organs-for-transplant. Again, and perhaps in much more critical ways than I have experienced in Ireland and the UK, the problems that are the focus of this book are human problems primarily—long before they have become anthropological problems—problems that require working through on an almost daily basis.

The insights and understandings that inform this book have been built up over time in conjunction and collaboration with others—patients, medical staff, medical suppliers, pharmacists, fellow researchers, friends, and colleagues. I wish to give recognition and thanks to these others here.

IN GRATITUDE

This book is the outcome of the participation of fifty-one patients, thirty-four family members—some of whom were donors and caregivers—sixteen doctors, seven social workers, seven nurses, one psychologist, one organ donation coordinator, one nutritionist, seven patient associations, four policy makers, five pharmaceutical and laboratory representatives, and one pharmacist—among scholars, researchers, and citizens too many to enumerate. Each and every one provided access to an unfamiliar world, connected up its elements and pointed out those critical features that lend substance and form to renal care and the technologies of transplant medicine.

My heartfelt thanks for the time you all have taken to work with me. In particular, I thank the families who feature prominently in this book and the extraordinary committed staff of the public hospital—where this ethnographic study unfolded. My sincere thanks to Dr. Guillermo Garcia Garcia and the nephrology staff in Guadalajara for their steadfast support for this project, for making it possible, and for their openness toward and acceptance of the ambiguities of anthropology.

I would never have ended up in Mexico and I would never have started this project if not for Dr. Franciso Mercado—a trained physician, anthropologist, and researcher at the University of Guadalajara—who sadly passed away earlier this year. His friendship, academic support and collegiality, good humor, and kindness ground the origins of this project.

Recognition and sincerest gratitude are owed to Cesar Padilla Altamira, the research assistant who worked with me, conducting interviews and observations. He has translated Mexico's political, social, and medical life for me and has taught me to see beyond the surface of everyday social interactions and into the richness of Mexican culture. He has read each chapter in this book and corrected my many mistakes and assumptions. Cesar's interest and commitment to issues of inequality in his home country have been an inspiration. I'm happy to say that this project furnished Cesar with a point of departure for his PhD. His own project focused on the challenges faced by uninsured Mexican dialysis patients who conduct and manage this replacement therapy within their homes. His beautifully crafted ethnographic study stands in direct conversation with this book.

Michael Mair, my friend and colleague, has been unwaveringly generous. Without him, I could not have seen the analytical possibilities that have shaped this book. He has introduced me to literatures I may not have otherwise read and ideas that have been foundational to my own academic path. I am most grateful for his sharing with me his thinking and reading on the sociology of the state—the subject of his forthcoming book *The Problem of the State*—and for reading countless versions of my chapters.

Kirsty Bell, fellow anthropologist, has been indispensable to the completion of this book, reading chapters, often at very short notice, offering intellectual, analytical, and editing guidance, and ensuring I kept to my deadlines. She has kept me focused and positive throughout and to her I owe a profound debt of thanks.

My brother Cahail Kierans, a talented graphic designer, has been of immense help in the selection and editing of all photos used and always responsive to last-minute requests.

I've had a number of very valuable opportunities to present different aspects of my analysis at seminars and symposiums. The challenging feedback and academic support I received have been instrumental to the final versions presented in the book. I am particularly grateful for invitations to talk from Pete Wade, Anthropology Department, University of Manchester; Sahra Gibbon, Anthropology Department, University College London; Bob Simpson and Tom Widger, Anthropology Department, Durham University; Mark McGuire, Anthropology Department, Maynooth University; Sabine Strasser, Anthropology Department, University of Bern. Other colleagues who have been indispensable to this project through their intellectual support and friendship are David Whyte and Nicole Vitellone, University of Liverpool; Jessie Cooper, City University, London; Jane Parish, Keele University; Eduardo Ibarra Hernandez, Universidad Autónoma San Luis Potosí, Mexico; Megan Crowley-Matoka, North Western University, Illinois, USA.

Philip McCormack, from Dublin, deserves the warmest of thanks for his calm and keen editorial eye when I needed a pair of fresh eyes at a given moment, but also for a constant supply of music that often helped me take a deep breath before getting back to work. Esperanza Avalos is the wonderful woman I stay with in Guadalajara—she is the rarest of people—and has been mother, sister, friend, confidant, and research informant, regaling me with local gossip, making me laugh, and helping me to see the city of Guadalajara in its more local and intimate guises.

My PhD students—Maria-Anne Moore, Stefanie Meysner, Julia Rehsmann, and Shelda Smith—have been a wonderful inspiration throughout the process of writing.

The production of this book and the ethnographic work that underpins it would not have been possible without financial and institutional support. I want to thank first and foremost—my academic home department—Public Health and Policy at the University of Liverpool and, in particular, Margaret Whitehead for her support and commitment to the importance of anthropological research and for supporting my sabbatical leave 2017–2018 to complete this book at the wonderful state library at Aarhus University; the Brocher Foundation, Geneva, Switzerland, for supporting and housing my writing fellowship in 2013; the Peter Lienhardt Memorial Fund, Oxford University, which funded my initial travel to Mexico, and the Wellcome Trust, UK, which funded later research travel and which has enabled me to continue my relationship with Mexico and transplant medicine. Additionally, this book has benefited considerably from the generous feedback of anonymous reviewers and Lenore Manderson's sharp eye.

Most personally, thank you to my family in Ireland: to Tommy, Molly, Cahail, Niamh, and Fergal—who have been my most enduring supports throughout and who have put up with infrequent journeys home, particularly at times of need for a close Irish family.

Finally, to my partner, Mads Sorensen, who has given me the best of all worlds, whose intellectual support, editorial insight, fun, laughter, cooking, love, and long walks through Denmark's beautiful landscape have sustained me through a long period of writing with minimum fuss and stress. Thank you for seeing me over all those final hurdles.

Ciara Kierans
MAY 2019, Aarhus and Liverpool

CHRONIC FAILURES

INTRODUCTION
Encountering Regimes of Renal Care:
The Crucible of Experience

On one hot July morning in 2011, I met four young people with failing or already failed kidneys. They were all in-patients, receiving various forms of renal care (medical care for kidney disease) in a Mexican public hospital. The hospital was widely known and well regarded as a hospital for poor and uninsured patients, many of whom travelled great distances to receive medical treatment there.

Carlos was the first kidney patient I met there. He was resting in a two-bed isolation ward, watching a small portable TV. The ward was at one end of the fifth-floor nephrology wing, located in a high rise concrete extension known as La Torre (The Tower).[1] From the small size of his frame, he looked about fourteen years old, but he was, in fact, twenty. He was recovering from transplant surgery after fifteen years of progressively worsening kidney disease, three of which had been spent shifting between peritoneal dialysis and hemodialysis treatments.[2] His mother and organ donor, Gloria, was recuperating in another ward on the floor below and appeared to be relaxed and in good spirits after her surgery. I was introduced to them both during morning ward rounds by Ana, one of the senior nephrologists. Ana wanted to see how they were doing and to pass on some left-over packets of prednisone for Carlos (prednisone is a synthetic corticosteroid drug used as part of immunosuppression therapy for transplant recipients). They were given to her by another patient who suffered kidney rejection after transplant surgery and no longer needed them.

Carlos and his mother were typical of the patients who were treated at the public hospital; they were members of a poor family who lived outside Mexico's social insurance system. They had no state entitlements to any form of renal care, which included organ transplantation and various forms of dialysis. To support her son's medical care, especially the recent organ transplant, Gloria invested great efforts in fundraising, appealing to friends, family, and local businesses for financial support. It was a struggle to amass enough money, and Carlos's father resorted to begging on the streets of Guadalajara, appealing to passers-by to help his son. Then the unexpected happened. A local TV channel, on hearing about their plight, agreed to act as a broker to find an appropriate benefactor to help fund the surgery, pre-transplant protocols, and the various physiological and psychological tests for both mother and son, as required prior to transplantation.

When I met Gloria and Carlos, a crew from the TV channel had already been with them for a number of weeks, conducting interviews for a series of special interest programs centered on their story. The programs would document their experiences before and after the surgery and chart the progress of mother and son. Transcripts from these interviews were provided to me by medical staff over the course of what was my first month of fieldwork. The interviews highlighted Gloria's desire to give her son a "second life"; her worries about whether she would be an appropriate match; the fears felt by mother and son about undergoing surgery; the possibility of having to wait for a deceased organ should this opportunity fail; their suffering over the past fifteen years; and the exorbitant costs they accrued trying to fund peritoneal dialysis, hemodialysis, medical consultations, medications, and so on. Once the transplant surgery was over, the local channel reported its success. The journalists emphasized the debt of gratitude Carlos felt toward his mother, the heartfelt appreciation of both mother and son for their medical team, and their wish to give thanks to God and, of course, the TV channel for helping to support the operation. While the TV program focused on Carlos's determination to live, it readily acknowledged the all-too-real risk that he could reject the new kidney. The priority for all involved, at this precious post-transplant point, was the critical need to raise more money to urgently cover the costs of cyclosporine, the immunosuppressant that Carlos would now need to take regularly to stop his body from rejecting his new kidney.

A few doors down the corridor from Carlos, in a slightly larger three-bed ward, Julio was resting, having just had emergency hemodialysis. The wards that July day were hot and humid, not helped by the large rectangular windows that looked out over a sprawling Guadalajara and that intensified the heat from the beating sun. Sitting beside Julio was his grandfather, mother, and father. They had come from Balcones del Cuatro, a working-class neighborhood on the outskirts of the city. The nephrology department's daily census recorded Julio's age as forty-five, but he was, in fact, twenty-two years old. Administrative errors such as these were not uncommon. Reconciling patient cases with the paper-work that followed them became part of the navigational undertaking of my ethnographic work.

Julio had been diagnosed with chronic kidney disease (CKD) the previous October (CKD involves a progressive loss of kidney function over time. There is no cure for it and patients with this condition will need some form of dialysis or a kidney transplant in order to survive). After experiencing what he described as intense fatigue and dizziness, he visited a local doctor who insisted he get to a hospital right away. Once there, he needed emergency dialysis. His family didn't know why their son had CKD but ventured two possible explanations: because he had been born prematurely at seven months and his kidneys had not developed properly; or because he had worked in a paint factory for five years prior to diagnosis, which perhaps had resulted in exposure to lead in the paint (lead is nephrotoxic). Despite his critical state of health, Julio was reluctant to start treatment:

> I didn't want dialysis, and thought to look for other possibilities—plants, herbs, teas . . . When I ate, I vomited, so I went to a healer in a village near where we live. He gave me some teas and told me to drink 1.5 liters of liquid a day. This helped me to eat more, but my blood pressure rose, my feet and my face swelled, and I could no longer walk and had to use a cane . . . In the last days, I produced lots of spittle, I felt like I was drowning . . . the water was filling my lungs. So in the end, I had no other choice but to take dialysis. When I was first brought into the ER (emergency room), the nurses told me I was nearly gone, that I could have had a heart attack.

Julio was fitted with a catheter in his abdomen in order to prepare for peritoneal dialysis (continuous ambulatory peritoneal dialysis [CAPD] for the vast majority of patient cases), he was given instructions on how to manage his diet, and he returned home. Some weeks later, after eating peaches, which are not permitted due to their levels of potassium, he became ill and was hospitalized again.[3] Repeat hospitalizations occurred regularly, as a result of the difficulty of coping with the constraints of maintaining a strict diet and ensuring optimum clinical conditions for performing peritoneal dialysis in the home. On this particular occasion, Julio had acquired peritonitis, an infection to which patients performing home dialysis are particularly vulnerable.[4] He had also been eating *tuna* (a fruit from the cactus, often referred to as prickly pear), which had again raised his potassium levels. Julio talked about how difficult he found his hospital visits, particularly the long waits in the ER and sleepless nights spent in the *salas* (the hospital's much older, traditional wards) surrounded by other sick and dying patients. Each time Julio came to the hospital, his family had to pay for everything—his hospitalization, dialysate solutions, medications, and so on. On this occasion, he needed a new catheter that would cost approximately 900 pesos (72 U.S. dollars; at time of fieldwork, 12.47 pesos = US$1.00).

As with every other patient and their family members who attend the public hospital, the financial and moral burden of CKD and its treatments, both in clinical and domestic settings, dominated our conversations. Julio was at pains to point out how much his family had to sacrifice for his health.

> At home, we had a small shop, a family business. Being on peritoneal dialysis meant that my mum could not work but had to take care of me instead. It also meant we

needed to use the shop as a space for my treatment and supplies. To prepare, we had to paint the room and put a new door on it. We were told we needed to use a special antibacterial oil paint to prevent mold—this all cost 4000 pesos [320 U.S. dollars]. We also had to buy a table, a new bed, a mattress, a lot of other materials, such as various tubes, face masks, gloves . . . [His father interrupts, "you forgot the silicone for the windows to keep out air, to keep out dirt . . . dust."] Yes, yes, it was all a big expense.

Apart from a few donated objects, such as a microwave oven given to him by his grandmother, the family resourced Julio's treatment by borrowing from neighbors and local money lenders.[5] This, of course, meant they incurred weekly repayments on top of all their other expenses. Furthermore, Julio explained, the family had very recently decided to start the protocols for transplantation on advice from their doctors. Julio's father, who had agreed to be his donor, stood up to hand me a piece of paper. On it was a list of laboratory tests and medical examinations Julio was obliged to take. His father explained that it was very important to him that he offer his kidney to his son. Some years back, he explained, he suffered a road accident and had sustained head injuries. He was left disabled for quite some time and Julio looked after him, as his main caregiver. For Julio's father, this was now his chance to reciprocate.

Next to Julio, in the same three-bed ward, Luis, another young man in his early twenties, twisted and turned as he struggled with leg cramps.[6] He was lying underneath a collection of religious pictures, prayers, and scapulars that his mother had carefully taped to the top of his bed.[7] She and Luis's father were sitting by his side. Up until his diagnosis, at the age of fifteen, Luis had worked with other members of his family as a farm laborer in the "berries" (multinational companies that cultivate and export berries to the United States). They worked and lived in one of the small villages that skirt Lake Chapala—Mexico's largest lake, approximately 60 kilometers outside Guadalajara. Like other families in the area, they were dependent both on the lake and local agri-companies for their livelihood.

Luis's family also did not know why he had CKD; neither did his doctors. Luis joked that it was because he drank too much Coca-Cola, an explanation readily given by patients and doctors alike for the rising number of Mexicans suffering from conditions like kidney disease and diabetes. Like other young, poor, and very often rural patients, Luis arrived at the hospital with kidneys too small to biopsy in order to establish a clear cause.[8] The fact that the causes of so many cases of CKD in Mexico are not known makes "unknown" an important category of reference for the condition.[9] It is referred to as the second most significant cause of CKD after diabetes. Ana explained that for people like Luis, who lived by Lake Chapala, there were growing concerns about the toxicity of the water but, to date, there was insufficient scientific evidence to link potential pollutants in the lake to people diagnosed with CKD.

Luis was brought to the hospital on 19 May 2011, only a few weeks prior to our meeting, and was put on intermittent dialysis, medication, and a new dietary regimen, his kidney function not yet in an "end stage." In describing the onset of his condition, he regarded his symptoms as unremarkable, saying, "I felt nothing. It happened during the summer, a few years ago. I walked to work as usual and felt nothing different. One day I asked for a rest day, as we had been working for several weeks and I was tired. We were going to burn pasture—it usually only takes three people, so I decided, why not ask for a day off. But on that day, I remember feeling very, very tired. My friends wanted to play tennis, but I had no desire to play, I was so tired."

Luis went on to describe how he later collapsed and his family had to get an ambulance to bring him to the emergency department. His mother interrupted, "This was so hard for us, it is because we have nothing. We had to ask many people for help to cover Luis's medications, to stay in the hospital, to pay for the tests." Luis went on to explain that they had to negotiate forcefully with the hospital's social workers to have their costs reduced, and to ask everyone they knew for money as well as using up what little the family could earn or had been able to save.[10] Luis's father said quietly, "I work so hard . . . all of the money is for him [Luis]. Sometimes, I am left with only 50 pesos for myself. Everything I have is for my son." Luis nodded in agreement and proceeded to talk about the difficulties of maintaining a new diet, one the entire household had to accommodate and endure, "Well, the diet is to eat vegetables, eat chicken but almost no broth, no salt, no fat, nothing like that . . . It's bland, but I'm getting used to it . . . My mum makes me fish fillet with vegetables in a tamale leaf. It's boring but I have to eat it." His mother nodded and interjected, "He is always hungry—it is a total change of food. He wants carnitas, tamales and chili, all the good things to taste. He can eat fish or chicken, some red meat but only twice a week . . . no pork, no salt, or garlic, no tomatoes. It's not just for him, it is a total change for the family and very, very expensive . . . what can we buy to eat? We can't just eat beans and tortillas."

Luis and his family had been in the hospital for almost three weeks when I met them. His mother stayed nearby at a religious hostel. His father, meanwhile, slept on the hospital ward floor beside his son. During the day, he went out to the small park directly in front of the hospital, carrying with him a piece of cardboard on which to lie and sleep in the sun. As I stood up to leave them, Luis's mother, in an effort to communicate something essential about living with this condition, said, "It's like . . . it makes us all work hard because we don't really know how to get around and do all these things. We're working hard constantly moving all the time, going here, going there. And when you don't know anything, you have to learn by force. It's a baptism by fire." The labor of sickness—the necessity of moving continually in search of care, learning how to mobilize resources and support, the unceasing effort to secure medical treatments—underpinned every conversation I had with family members and patients within the hospital.

At the end of that particular morning of ward visits, Ana explained that a mother and daughter had just arrived to prepare for transplant surgery. This was scheduled for the following day. As there were no beds available yet, and as both had little to do but wait, she said they were amenable to talking. Ana stressed that it was important to understand their circumstances and experiences thus far. They were waiting in the white bucket seats between the lifts and the fifth-floor wards, but I could interview them in one of the two small work-rooms generally used by medical staff. I had been given a key and the freedom to use one of these rooms anytime I came to the hospital. Of the two rooms, the larger was always busy, used mostly by nurses and junior doctors to print out the morning patient census, have impromptu meetings, catch up on paperwork, eat lunch, and so on. The second one was smaller, quieter, and, for the most part, used by hospital consultants and senior staff. It was simply equipped, containing a long table, eight chairs, some shelves, and cabinets. It had a disorderly collection of documents stacked in arbitrary heaps and numerous cardboard boxes full of patient files. The room had a small computer tucked into a corner, but it was not networked and only occasionally used. The doctors, in any case, carried smart phones or laptops with them, and worked as they moved throughout the hospital. This room, like everywhere else in the nephrology ward, suffered the July heat. Its only window, when opened, let in the noise of the city, so it remained closed; a large, droning fan provided whatever relief it could. It was, moreover, only a quasi-private space, frequently interrupted by patients, family members, nurses, cleaning staff, and pharmaceutical reps, among others.

Alicia and her mother Teresa—kidney recipient and donor—came into the room carrying a large, striped, waxed shopping bag full of hospital files, notes, clinical histories, and drug prescriptions, among other odds and ends of patient information: an entire medical history of a CKD case crammed into a makeshift archive. Teresa pulled out a folder that contained all the results of their pre-transplant protocols, for example, blood and tissue matching tests and psychological assessments. They were to be given to Ana, but as she had slipped out to check on another patient, Teresa passed them straight to me. I respectfully glanced at the *historia clínica* (clinical history), which stated that Teresa, the donor and mother, was thirty-four years old, divorced, a non-smoker and a non-drinker who had been rated as having a "good psychological orientation" to donating a kidney to her daughter.

She immediately started to talk through the various tests they had undergone in preparation for the next day's surgery. Eighteen-year-old Alicia sat quietly in her beige-colored tracksuit, her long hair tied back in a ponytail. She kept her eyes fixed on the table and fiddled with her jewelry. Given that a research interview, however informal, had not been planned, and was far from their immediate priority, both were agreeable to it. Teresa explained that Alicia had suffered many problems. Initially, she was on peritoneal dialysis, but due to recurring infections and problems with the catheter, she was told she would need hemodialysis. She couldn't be accommodated at the public hospital due to limited space, and so had to attend a private clinic run by PiSA, a Mexican pharmaceutical company. Dialysis there cost 1,100 pesos per session (88 U.S. dollars). This was a reduced price, one Alicia's doctors at the public hospital helped to negotiate. As Alicia had already started the protocols for transplantation, it was expected that she would not remain on dialysis for long. This was something she was counting on, having found it difficult to comply with restrictions to her diet. However, on this particular day, what was foremost on the minds of mother and daughter was where they would find the money for the immunosuppressants Alicia would need after surgery, should it be successful.

Alicia and her mother came from a poor neighborhood called Mesa Colorada, north of Zapopan, part of the wider metropolitan area of Guadalajara. Teresa worked there as an *empleada doméstica* (a maid) and had been with the same family for fifteen years. She felt fortunate that her employer was a nurse and sensitive to her daughter's condition. However, because Teresa had to work, Alicia came to all her hospital appointments alone. She explained,

> At first it was hard, but now the whole hospital is my second home. I feel glad that my mum can give me her kidney, because I know other patients like me who have no-one to give them a kidney and they are like waiting corpses. But we have gone through so many bad things. It is hard without money. At least we have some support, thank God. I don't know what will happen today—or when a bed will be ready or if we will be able to stay together or if I have to wait in the *salas*. I have had some very sad stays in the *salas*—I was there once on Christmas Day, when the lady beside me died. Everyone was crying.

Teresa and Alicia had little financial support from their family, although Teresa's ex-husband helped out from time to time. To cover the costs of medical care, Teresa appealed to various governmental and non-governmental agencies. Much of Alicia's dialysis-related costs as well as their combined pre-transplant protocols and tests were covered by Desarrollo Integral de la Familia (DIF), a state-funded organization that supports families in need, and Caritas, the international Catholic charity. Teresa explained,

> It has been very difficult, because we don't have the economic means. This is a very expensive disease, very expensive, and I need to go asking for support. DIF helped with hemodialysis. Each session cost 1,100 pesos [88 U.S. dollars] and Alicia had to do two a week. I thank God because they have helped me for eight months. With the protocols and tests needed for the transplant, this has been very difficult. In November 2010, we did all the necessary tests, but then had no money to pay for the surgery, so we had to stop everything. The doctors looked to see if they could

help us through Seguro Popular but they couldn't.[11] At that time, the price of transplant surgery was 15,400 pesos [1,235 U.S. dollars], but there are rumors that it could rise to 73,000 pesos [5,854 U.S. dollars].

All I want is for Alicia to have a more stable life, because she is the only child I have ... and because, as the doctors told us, this is to have a new life, not a normal life, but a more stable life. That is why I was determined to donate a kidney—to give her a more stable life.

THE PUBLIC HOSPITAL

Alicia, Carlos, Luis, and Julio were all patients of Antiguo Hospital Civil, a Mexican public hospital that has looked after families like theirs—the poor of Jalisco—for over 200 years.[12] It was founded in 1792 by Fray Antonio Alcalde, a man already in his seventies when he arrived in Nueva Galicia, today Guadalajara, a city that at that time was ravaged by epidemics and famine. Its reputation as a hospital for the poor continues today, as patients travel across the state of Jalisco and beyond in search of care. They come with conditions such as cancers, diabetes, HIV—very different from those first treated there—alongside the persistent infectious diseases that have not relinquished their grip on the country's impoverished classes. Chronic, so-called non-communicable diseases intertwine with older forms of suffering, bound together by histories of poverty and inequality, most recently tied to the growth of Mexico's towns and cities that have provided little refuge or economic opportunity for the rural and indigenous migrant.

The hospital, situated adjacent to the historic cemetery Panteón de Belen, is nestled among the faded grandeur of Guadalajara's low-rise and congested city streets. Here, run-down *tapatian* houses, houses typical of downtown Guadalajara, sit within a thriving local economy of food markets, family restaurants, street vendors, mobile phone shops, medical suppliers, pharmacies, and laboratories, all woven into the fabric of hospital life. This bustling neighborhood is but a few short blocks from the city's historic center—a grand plaza furnished by colonial governmental buildings, churches, galleries, theaters, and fountains. Here, in the early-nineteenth century, Miguel Hidalgo, a Catholic priest and leader of the Mexican war of independence, signed his proclamation to end slavery. Today, Mexico's second city is home to five million inhabitants. Although it stands as a progressive, cosmopolitan, and commercial city, its historical, economic, and cultural past still resonates in the city's built environment, its social and ethnically diverse population, and the inequalities that mark out their differences. Guadalajara today still reflects a Mexico, described by Alexander von Humboldt in 1811, as a country of inequality. "Nowhere does there exist such a fearful difference in the distribution of fortune, civilization, cultivation of the soil, and population. . . . The capital and several other cities have scientific establishments, which will bear

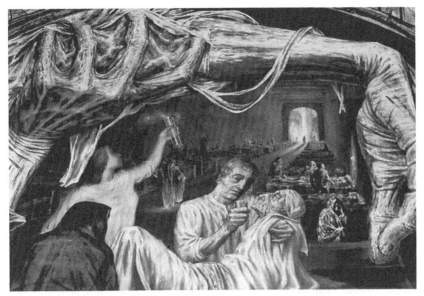

FIGURE 1. A small section of Flores's mural *La Historia de la Medicina,* depicting the *salas* in the nineteenth century.

a comparison with those of Europe. The architecture of the public and private edifices, the elegance of the furniture, the equipages, the luxury and dress of the women, the tone of society, all announce a refinement to which the nakedness, ignorance, and vulgarity of the lower people form the most striking contrast" (von Humboldt in Cordera and Tello 2015 [1984], 7).

This mix of the historical and contemporary is reflected in the hospital's architecture and in the continuities and discontinuities that have assembled themselves through it. Its colonial inheritance is on display at the main entrance, which opens up into a series of beautifully kept courtyard gardens and open-air corridors supported by arched colonnades. In this section of the hospital, the original *salas* (hospital wards) have been preserved, each named after former physicians memorialized for their respective roles in the hospital's history.[13] The *salas,* a series of long-roomed, sixty-bed wards, extend outward in panoptic fashion from a round central foyer, which, at one time, housed the nurses' station. Today, the space is unused save as a crossroads for staff and patients making their way between the old and the new. The walls and ceiling of the foyer are arched and vaulted and covered completely in murals depicting *La Historia de la Medicina,* a local history of medicine set in the context of Mexican and Jaliscan political change and poverty (see a photograph of a small fragment of the mural in figure 1). They were painted in 1993 by the Guadalajara-born painter and muralist Gabriel Flores, an artist whose work depicting Mexican history can be seen throughout the city's government buildings and educational institutions.

Many patients spend their first few nights in the *salas* before moving to specialist wards as and when beds are made available. The *salas*, although providing greatly needed space, have little of the relative comfort and quiet of the newer wards in La Torre, one of the hospitals more recent medical wings. Younger patients are placed alongside elderly patients; acute patients alongside those who are chronically ill and dying. This is a traumatic introduction to the hospital, particularly for the young renal patients whose condition announces itself suddenly and with little warning. At the end furthest from the hospital's entrance, the *salas* feed into what were once the hospital's lecture halls and teaching rooms, pedagogical spaces where patients could easily be wheeled out for inspection as teaching aids. The doctors who are now based in this part of the building manage the complex incongruities of sickness and suffering that fold back onto these long histories of social suffering, while simultaneously being refracted via twenty-first century social, cultural, and technical forces.

These tensions are also clear in the flow of funds to the hospital. Hospital Civil is a large tertiary facility supported by the Secretaria de Salud Jalisco (SSJ, Ministry of Health of Jalisco) and is financed by state and federal funds, private donations, and contributions from non-governmental organizations. It functions as an independent healthcare provider with its own budget and board of directors. Patients are charged a negotiated fee according to level of income. Its status as a hospital for the poor notwithstanding, this is not an institution that is easy to access, particularly for those without means. Its various entrances and exits are tightly controlled by security guards who ensure that those who enter have the required documentation and appointments. As the hospital also serves the local prison population, armed guards are part of the daily and differentiated personnel who frequent it. They arrive in paramilitary gear, often six to a handcuffed prisoner, flanking them on all sides, briskly clearing hallways so that prisoners can be marched to their appointments. As a non-Mexican in this setting, I evaded such scrutiny and policing. Few would question my right to be there, and most would assume I was medical staff, an international doctor who had come for research or training. Nevertheless, to prevent scrutiny as I came into the hospital in the mornings, I was told to purchase a doctor's white coat; together with a researcher identity card, which I wore on my lapel, this gave me the capacity to enter, exit and move as I pleased.[14]

For those who needed help most, the situation was very different. From very early morning, patients and their families gathered outside the hospital's walls, forming large queues, and marking out all-too-visible zones of inclusion and exclusion. Accompanying family members were often left to wait along the perimeter roads and walls, and in the small green park to the front of the hospital. They were a ready-made clientele for the vast informal army of vendors selling food, second-hand clothes, electrical gadgets, herbal medicines, and countless Catholic goods. Once inside the hospital, time was spent waiting: for appointments, for beds, for social workers, for test results, and so on. As the outpatients' department was in the throes of reconstruction, those attending waited outside a temporary prefabricated unit, directly behind La Torre. They sat on walls, on plastic chairs, or under the shade of the few small trees that survived within the grounds of the hospital. A large sign "asked" for cooperation and understanding. The ubiquitous regulation of access reflects what Javier Auyero calls the persuasion of the destitute of the need to be patient. Waiting, as a form of stratification, "one of the ways of experiencing the effects of power" (Auyero 2011, 5), was all too clear in this setting.

Forms of stratification, implicit and explicit, characterize the public hospital, which also functions as a large teaching hospital under the institutional governance of the University of Guadalajara. Both university and hospital are formally and informally embedded in the wider political governance structures of the city and are widely felt to have little autonomy outside of the city's religious and political institutions. At times, it seemed as if there were more junior doctors moving between corridors than patients, and, for many of those who came to it as part of their medical training, the hospital would be little more than a step on the way to larger medical institutions and specialist hospitals treating, perhaps, a different type or class of Mexican patient.

FIELDWORK AND THE GUIDED CHARACTER OF UNDERSTANDING

The public hospital was a requisite first step for this ethnographic inquiry rather than the discrete site of fieldwork. It was where I began to trace the various routes taken by those who moved through its emergency rooms, surgical theaters, and hospital wards—Mexico's poor and uninsured—and the condition which afflicted them—CKD. Neither patient nor condition were bound to or by the hospital. Both leaked out into the world, to the streets around the hospital, to neighborhoods, homes and villages, and much farther beyond still. The hospital was less locus than nexus in the flow of patients, information, and all manner of health-related things. The various routes patients and their families took intersected a political economy. In doing so, they pulled into view the welfare state arrangements through which uninsured patients acquired a social status and access to treatment.

In the hospital, I became acquainted with the challenging character of CKD and the regimes of renal care it depended on, in particular various modes of dialysis and transplantation. It was also clear, from the outset, that I was encountering something quite different to what I had experienced in my previous work in Ireland and in the UK. During my first week of fieldwork, I was told by one of the nephrologists, "We want you to see how bad things are here . . . Mexico is the opposite of countries like the UK. No transplant program there would start without appropriate funding. Here we start and rely on the fact that money will be raised as time goes on, but it is the patients who have to pay for everything, hospital stays, prescriptions, accessories for CAPD, drugs to fight infections ... everything."

Efforts made to show how "bad things were" were central to helping make the unfamiliar familiar. This began with an invitation to attend morning ward rounds and sit in on consultations so that introductions could be made to staff and patients alike. I was repeatedly told by Ana, one of the consultant nephrologists, "This is our reality; you *have to* understand our reality." Her initial strategy for providing entry to this reality, for coming at it from within, was to guide me and Cesar Padilla-Altamira (the research assistant working on this project) through the morning "census" or daily in-patient list: a one-page printout containing a patient's name, age, stage of renal failure, treatment modality, reason for hospitalization, and room number.

Establishing contact with patients and their families in the hospital was not difficult. One resource they all had in abundance was time, time otherwise spent waiting for beds, for test results, to see their doctors, to meet with social workers, and so on. Waiting was also an integral part of the labor of sickness. That said, I was profoundly aware that most patients and their families had little choice *but* to talk to us, to entertain our questions, despite all assurances they were not obliged to. Their vulnerability and their need to secure care for their loved ones created few options but to comply with their doctors' requests to give us a little of their time too. Though not always optimum, ward rounds provided an initial route to meeting patients and their families, observe institutional practice, and follow the work of doctoring. They also provided an opportunity to organize further interviews outside of clinical settings. Tracing the contours of renal care outward, we followed it into kinship and community settings, places in which its social and technical arrangements extended. Renal care inevitably placed a burden on women, whose commitment to their loved ones was already an extension of engrained, gendered histories of caring. By slowly working outward from the hospital to the various sites co-implicated or imbricated with it, CKD also produced an awkward symbiosis between kidney transplantation and the modalities of dialysis upon which it depends. In Mexico, peritoneal dialysis—by far the most common modality used—reflects the various ways in which the specific practices of medicine are circumscribed by the limitations of a profoundly fragmented healthcare system. I explore this in some detail in the chapters which follow.

The setting for my first tentative encounters with the specificities of transplant medicine and renal care, more generally, was the fifth floor of the public hospital. The fifth floor was in a separate wing of the hospital called La Torre, a relatively recent nine-story modern extension to this two-hundred-year-old public hospital. The hospital had grown slowly into a series of extensions, its redevelopments and new wings all linked by an internal constellation of corridors and pathways that gave some coherence to an otherwise disparate collection of architectural styles and functional spaces (Hull 2012b). The fifth floor was accessed by elevators, which always seemed full, and Ana, more often than not, took the narrow stairway that zig-zagged up the back of the building, the passing of each floor marked by a walk past a solitary and often out-of-order public toilet.

The fifth floor was the main site of activity for nephrology. It comprised a succession of small one-, two-, and three-bedroom patient wards—with capacity for approximately thirty-five to forty patients. It also had a small surgical theater, regularly used for fitting catheters in patients preparing for peritoneal dialysis—a room that doubled-up as a training space for caregivers of these same patients. Beyond these rooms were a number of stock rooms for supplies and medications, staff meeting rooms, a nurses' station, a small religious grotto, and a room with a double-set of bunk beds and a bathroom for staff on night duty. Outside the main door into the fifth-floor wards, on the landing area between the elevators and the back stairwell was a small makeshift waiting area. In the mornings it was cramped and crowded with family members and patients, most waiting for beds to become available. Those who had a seat sat quietly and patiently. Those who were sick and fatigued took blankets and slept on the floor in the few small spaces that didn't block the movement of medical staff and trolleys.

One particular morning, when making my way onto the fifth floor, I stood behind two doctors trying to push, shove, and cajole a trolley full of dialysate solution in through the main doorway to the ward. One turned to me—and said with irony, "This is Mexico! I wish there was a politician here to see us now. I would tell him, look we have so many resources, we cannot get them all through the door." The rhetoric of inadequate resourcing and the invocation of political or state culpability would be repeated mantra-like in the course of hospital visits and interviews. These responses, however, only inadequately conveyed what I came to see was the deeper, more finely grained politics of healthcare at work in the operation of the hospital, as I will discuss in later chapters.

The fifth floor in no way met the demand for beds, so renal patients often found themselves distributed throughout the hospital, moving between the *salas* and the newer clinical wards, when space could be negotiated or simply taken. The politics of resourcing—as an everyday set of practical considerations, decisions, and commitments between the state and its sick citizens—provided me with the analytical space to think both within and beyond the Mexican case. It provided a starting point from which to document and understand access to technological care outside of welfare arrangements; the various ways in which sick bodies acquire visibility or recede from systems of governance and administration; the spread of new markets in healthcare through technoscientific developments; and their capacity to produce health or deny it. I want to suggest that what the staff and patients in these opening descriptions were directing my attention to was not an essential distinction between European medical systems and the situation in Mexico, but the problem of specificity. What I took from my fieldwork in Mexico is a key lesson: whenever we look at technologies like organ transplantation and forms of dialysis, we must look at the ways in which they elaborate specific forms of biopolitics.[15]

FOCUS AND CONTRIBUTION OF THIS BOOK

The problematic ethics, politics, and economics of organ exchange commonly foreshadow our engagements with it. When placed into a Mexican context, these concerns are coupled with presuppositions of corruption, violence, and illegality. When discussing my project with others, academics and non-academics alike, it was readily assumed I was motivated by the dark or illicit side of organ transplantation. I found myself repeatedly having to explain what this book was *not* about: that it was not about an illegal or underground trade in organs; that it was not about organ theft; nor indeed about medical tourism and the commodification of poor bodies for consumption by rich bodies. Important, relevant, and critical as these issues are, attending to them can serve to sensationalize and exceptionalize aspects of transplant medicine, while turning a blind eye to the more mundane and unexceptional—but no less problematic or scandalous—aspects of healthcare access. As a consequence, this book is about CKD and the biotechnical treatments it relies on, lived out in the context of poverty, inequality, and uneven welfare arrangements. It is about the labor that is required and the necessary routes patients have to follow to secure access to treatment. These routes to care are normalized, bureaucratically, socially, and epidemiologically, and turned into a locus for exploitation and profit. My goal throughout this book is to locate sickness, poverty, and healthcare within the political economy that generates their specific expressions and prospects and to show that technologized medicine, in the context of a chronic condition like CKD, is a critical site for exploring the situated elaboration of contemporary biopolitics in Mexico, as elsewhere.

CKD is on the rise. It is an urgent concern, not only for Mexico but for countries the world over. Once considered a disease of affluence, linked to urbanization and sedentary lifestyles, it is today a critical global public health problem, disproportionately impacting the world's poorest citizens. Approximately 500 million people are thought to suffer from CKD globally (Stanifer et al. 2016), with the majority—80 percent—living in low- and middle-income countries (Bello et al. 2017). The 2015 Global Burden of Disease Study positioned CKD as the twelfth most common cause of death, accounting for 1.1 million deaths worldwide (Murray et al. 2016). Over the last ten years, mortality rates from CKD have increased by 31.7 percent, making it one of the fastest-rising causes of death alongside diabetes and dementia (Lange Neuen et al. 2017). In Mexico, the prevalence of CKD among the poor is two to three times higher than among the general population, made worse by poor access to health insurance and to timely and appropriate healthcare (Garcia-Garcia and Jha 2015). CKD is far from a discrete condition. Its complex etiologies show it to be an outcome of other conditions, which include diabetes, hypertension, glomerulonephritis, vascular diseases, polycystic kidney disease, pharmacological substance use, and various types of trauma and injury. Type 2 diabetes is formally established as the leading cause of CKD, itself understood as constituting a global pandemic. Like diabetes, CKD is readily explained as a condition precipitated by so-called lifestyle or behavioral factors, which in turn have served to individualize and de-politicize the condition (Montoya 2011).

The causal story of CKD, however, has begun to change. This is because a new variant of the condition has emerged that pulls social and structural concerns, as opposed to individual and behavioral concerns, more firmly into view. Over the past twenty years, across Central America and Southeast Asia in particular, there has been an unexplained increase and change in the etiological profile of CKD. This new variant has been classified as chronic kidney disease of unknown origin (CKDu) or, in the case of Central America, Mesoamerican nephropathy (MeN) (Correa-Rotter, Wesseling, and Johnson 2014). MeN, as the acronym indicates, is characterized by gender imbalances, estimated to have caused the premature death of at least 20,000 men within the region, the majority agricultural workers (Ramirez-Rubio et al. 2013). At its most extreme, the town of Chichigalpa, in Nicaragua, has seen CKDu claim close to 75 percent of all male deaths within a ten-year period, the majority of whom worked as sugarcane cutters at the Ingenio San Antonio sugar plantation, the largest in the country (Weiner et al. 2013). An expanding public health literature describes CKDu as a new global health problem for those living in the global south. Commonly referred to as a medical enigma, CKDu cannot be accounted for in conventional etiological terms—that is, attributed to established causes such as diabetes or hypertension—but instead is variously linked to social, cultural, and environmental factors. In Mexico, where concerns about the condition have only recently surfaced, CKDu is similarly considered to affect a young demographic, is associated with informal, precarious work (such as in the agri-industries, fishing, and mining), long-term environmental harm and degradation (Cárdenas-González et al. 2016), and with a political economy driven by NAFTA (North Atlantic Free Trade Agreement) and an impoverished regulatory environment. Those most affected by it tend to be from poor communities, often working with pesticides, and/or in the context of heavy metal pollution and contaminated water supplies (Wesseling, Crowe, and Hogstedt 2013). In contexts defined by unequal, metered access to healthcare, those who are poor are among those least likely to be able to pay for its treatments. High rates of CKDu in Mexico have been reported across the states of Aguascalientes, San Luis Potosi, Jalisco, Veracruz, and Tlaxcala (Cardenas-González et al. 2016).

That we have come to identify and learn about the spread of CKDu at all is in large part due to the efforts of those affected by it rather than any functional official monitoring and registry systems. The Nicaraguan sugar cane workers were the first to bring the problem to global attention through the establishment of La Asociación Chichigalpa por la Vida (ASOCHIVIDA)—the Chichigalpan Association for Life. Through it, they formally complained to the World Bank, a funder of the plantation, stating that workers were falling chronically ill due to the working conditions and practices of the plantation. ASOCHIVIDA embarked on sustained public demonstrations to demand recognition of and solutions to their suffering, raising attention globally to the ways in which kidney failure was decimating the working lives of men (Wright 2016). In Jalisco, by comparison, and as I will discuss later in the book, awareness of the disease has been less localized and more broadly linked to the structural conditions of poverty and environmental degradation.

Attempts to understand the rise and spread of this new variant of CKD are further complicated by the fact that the kidneys—the physiological site of the condition—tend to be so shriveled when patients present to doctors that they are difficult to biopsy and thus provide little traction for diagnosis. Furthermore, conventional diagnostics for kidney disease such as blood pressure measurement or dipstick urinalysis have poor sensitivity for detecting cases. This means that there are practical limits to ascertaining the percentage of CKD deaths that can actually be classified as CKDu, a situation made worse in Mexico by a fragmented healthcare system where patient data is not routinely shared and public health monitoring is partial. Nevertheless, a recent Mexican study describing the epidemiological characteristics of CKD in the country shows that CKD with an unknown etiology is on the increase, particularly among younger patients. Using data extrapolated over a twenty-year period (1994–2014) from Mexico's largest kidney transplantation program, an Instituto Mexicano de Seguro Social (IMSS)-affiliated program in Jalisco, the etiology of 80 percent of patient cases was classified as unknown.[16] Results were grouped into four five-year periods, showing that instances of CKDu increased from 67 percent of CKD cases in the first five-year period to 86 percent in the last. The figures are cause for alarm. As the majority of these patients are under the age of forty, and Mexico (represented by registry data collected by the states of Morelos and Jalisco) is already ranked first in incidence of CKD in the world (Solis-Vargas, Evangelista-Carrillo, and Puetes-Camacho 2016), the growing problem of kidney failure will place an already stressed healthcare system under more pressure.

The category 'unknown' is intriguing, problematic, and to some extent misleading. To be understood, it has to be seen in the context of what is assumed to be "known": the conventional causal story of CKD told via already established risk factors, such as diabetes, hypertension, glomerulonephritis in conjunction with obesity, sedentary lifestyles, and so on. Storying CKD in this way masks the fact that despite very well-established associations, these root conditions are also bound to etiological unknowns. Diabetes, itself, for example, as the anthropologist

Michael Montoya has shown, also occurs at an unstable confluence of biological, environmental, and social concerns. The conventional emphasis on risk factors, he contends, narrows our focus and "results in the erasure of the socioeconomic, historical and political contexts of populations affected by disease" (Montoya 2011, 87). CKDu throws these contexts starkly into relief and situates kidney disease as a fundamental problem of political economy, urging attention to what Sherine Hamdy (2012) has referred to as the political etiology of kidney disease.

During fieldwork in 2011 and 2012, CKDu had not acquired a great deal of attention from researchers and clinicians in Mexico. However, in the course of writing this book (2013–2018), this had started to change. Nonetheless, many of the patients whose accounts feature in this book had an uncertain diagnosis. They did not know why their kidneys had failed and neither did their doctors. What CKDu helps us to see is that kidney disease and the regimes of medical care bound up with it—a socio-medical problem and its biotechnical solutions—are formed out of the same basic stuff, emerging and gaining whatever measure of solidity and permanence they possess under the same sets of political and economic conditions. The articulation of one is the articulation of the other. Far from separate, discrete, or temporally related as cause to effect, as the origin myth suggests, they are instead co-eval and linked in processes of co-elaboration. Put most simply, as our knowledge and understanding of one increase, so does our knowledge and understanding of the other. What is more, both reflect the specific contexts within which this co-elaboration unfolds: they are, as I will show, not just context-sensitive but also context-saturated phenomena.

In this context of increasing global economic insecurity, the rising incidence of CKD and the entrenchment of commodified healthcare, I critically examine the implications of the articulation, growth, and spread of what I refer to as *regimes of renal care* and the complex of biotechnical treatments it relies on (see chapter 1 for discussion). These treatments are the situated and articulated arrangements of and forms of access to dialysis and transplant medicine—technoscientific domains that feed off and feed back into the challenges of our time. These technoscientific domains are reproduced and extended through processes of haphazard adaptation, accommodation, and localization rather than by following an invariant blueprint or core schematic passed down from some putative central architect. As a consequence, their local realizations—the forms they take in different national healthcare systems—are marked as much by the unique pathways through which they operate locally as by the characteristics they share in common. With organ transplantation the preferred treatment for CKD, and CKD increasing at alarming rates, this technoscientific regime continues to grow and spread. The question is how, with what implications, and for whom?

I take up these questions in this book via an ethnographic case, one that teaches us how to look beyond its own particular configurations. I do so by focusing on the specific ways uninsured patients access resource-intensive transplant medicine and forms of dialysis in Mexico, and the local production of different, intersecting, and often mutually interfering forms of medical "care" around them. I show how the connections between technological renal care, life, and power emerge as urgent "matters of concern" (Latour 2004) in the context of Mexico's predominantly living-related transplant program, by documenting the complex moves kidney patients with no form of social protection or welfare have to make in order to become eligible for dialysis and transplantation. These are Mexico's poor, approximately 50 percent of the country's population.

Without a visible or coherent logic of healthcare access, negotiating the arrangements of transplant medicine and other renal replacement therapies has catastrophic consequences for those with the least resources to expend in that effort. In carrying the costs (moral, social, and economic) and the burden of responsibility for care, the practices of poor patients and their families offer a critical vantage point from which to assess the dynamic interplay between the state, markets in healthcare, and the sick body—the terrain of biopolitics in the context of biotechnical interventions. In a global context of widening inequality, the Mexican case has particular significance because it shows how these sick bodies function simultaneously as sites for technoscientific differentiation and the production of surplus value. As a result, social divisions are not just reproduced, but reinforced, intensified, and extended by the consolidation of regimes of renal care, with people having to adapt to the needs of technologized medicine, whatever the substantial costs, rather than technologized medicine having to adapt to them. Although these processes are far from restricted to Mexico alone, but are at work the world over, in Mexico they can be seen with a clarity they do not always display elsewhere. Mexican society is characterized by profound social and health inequalities, divisions that have been amplified rather than ameliorated by ongoing waves of political and economic reform and the changes they have set in motion. Today, among OECD (Organisation for Economic Co-operation and Development) countries, Mexico records the largest inequalities in household income (OECD 2017). As a mixed corporatist/neoliberal welfare state (Esping-Andersen 1990), the country provides a vital lens for examining what happens when healthcare is reconfigured and made primarily accessible via the "cash nexus." The marked increased in CKD and the complex developments that are driving it are part of the elaboration of new biopolitical landscapes. These processes are intensifying worldwide and the Mexican case shows us their operation in a particularly stark form.

As the Mexican case helps us to see, if CKD is a disease that is emblematic of the social, political, and economic relations of our time, then organ replacement therapies are emblematic of the medicine of our time. Both, I will argue, are profoundly misunderstood. Although medical anthropologists, in particular, have begun the work of interrogating transplant medicine's differential articulations, they have rarely extended these to the comparative analysis of the heterogeneous biopolitical arrangements within which it is embedded. An analysis of that kind, however, must start by acknowledging the equivocal character of transplant medicine. Rather than accept the claims that arise regarding organ transplantation's status as a morally worthy therapeutic project, I attend to its disruptive and damaging influence on the very people it is meant to help, alongside its positive potentials.

In this book, I trace outward from the Mexican case to show how the technological modalities of renal care encountered by Mexican CKD patients constitute a global project with variable local configurations. These configurations help establish new forms of politics, economics, labor, and welfare in the way they put bodies and populations to work. A composite of parts, regimes of renal care implicate us all through global systems of economic and exchange relations, knowledge production and dissemination infrastructures, international networks of medical and scientific personnel, the remodeling of interpersonal relationships, and so on. What is important to the unfolding narrative of this book are the specific ways in which the different aspects of renal care are elaborated across various sites and settings over time, with new developments absorbed, altered, and made to work or fail. Extending anthropological insights, in this book I suggest we need to look at renal replacement therapies in a different way. Sick bodies are dependent on them and need access to them, but equally, transplant medicine and forms of dialysis are dependent on the labor of sick bodies to work. The Mexican case is of critical importance in this regard because the character of this dependency, and the work and elaboration which sustains it, are made particularly visible.

Based on ethnographic field research conducted during 2011, 2012, 2016, and 2017 in the central Mexican state of Jalisco, *Chronic Failures: Kidneys, Regimes of Care, and the Mexican State* advances a vital analysis of the workings of resource-intensive medical technologies in the context of a poorly resourced but highly (bio)politicized setting. The book has much to teach us about how transplant medicine and forms of dialysis work, not only in Mexico. The Mexican case provides an urgent lens on "all our futures," by showing what happens when technical interventions are disembedded from social structures of welfare and entitlement.[17] In doing so, this book echoes Biehl and Petryna's (2013) call for a concerted focus on the social, political, and economic processes associated with new paradigms in global health and on integrated approaches that recognize the profound interdependence of health, economics, government, and systems of social, political, and human rights. While explicitly building on existing bodies of scholarship across anthropology, science studies, and global health, I move such scholarship in new directions by making a number of theoretical interventions into our study of the biopolitical grounds of contemporary medicine-state-market relations. Primarily, I rethink analyses that cast organ replacement technologies as expressions of broad political and economic forces, such as neoliberalism and the processes of commoditization, to show instead how these biotechnical domains are also productive or give rise to such forces and the social relations that underpin them. I want to show that, in being used to extend life, these technologies both *have* and *make* politics.

OVERVIEW OF BOOK

The structure of this book is informed by the routes to care taken by uninsured Mexican kidney patients, and the particular manner in which they make visible interconnections between the state, market, and medicine as they converge on CKD; in other words, a political economy of renal care.

Chapter 1, "Studying Regimes of Renal Care," sets out the methodological ground of the book by asking: what is it we are faced with when we encounter regimes of renal care and their biotechnical arrangements; how do we go about studying them and what resources are required to do so? I explicitly draw on the idea of "regimes" to point out that the particular forms of intervention bound to CKD are neither fixed nor universal but have stabilized over time as culturally and institutionally recognized ways of organizing treatment and care. By focusing on those seeking out renal care—patients and their families, and the journeys they take, I show that it is in following them and their various engagements with organ replacement technologies, that we are taken to the many sites (social, political, and economic) within and across which renal care regimes are articulated and that generate arbitrary outcomes leading to harm and dispossession. In this chapter, I question commonly held assumptions about the stability of organ transplantation as a particular kind of cultural and medical object—in particular, its acquired status as *the* optimum mode of treatment for those suffering from CKD. Emphasizing the varied ways in which transplant medicine and the technological work bound up with it are made to function across different sites and settings, I reflect on what it means to treat organ transplantation as an object of ethnographic inquiry, drawing attention to the particular manner in which transplant medicine produces itself under different circumstances and acquires its status as a technological advance.

Following this, in chapter 2, "Biopolitics and the Analytics of a Population on the Move," I demonstrate the particular character of the biopolitical at play in Mexico and, in doing so, I make an important contribution to theorizing on this topic. I describe how the uneven development of transplant medicine in the context of the increasing burden of CKD in Mexico is the embodiment of a society deeply fractured by its own political economy. I detail the fragmented and complex organization of health service access, and the country's repeated efforts at healthcare reform. Seguro Popular (Popular Health Insurance), Mexico's most recent attempt to universalize healthcare, has failed to support CKD or its treatments. This is an initiative that is caught between the competing demands for universal coverage and market-driven approaches to healthcare provision. While these concerns resonate with similar challenges faced by other countries, Hospital Civil and its key protagonists acquire a particular significance: notably, the doctors who routinely work across public and private healthcare contexts and the patients and their families who continually move back and forth between them. Hospital Civil, and those whose paths crisscross within it, are presented as critical intermediaries in the flow of bodies, technology, and care.

By way of illustration, this chapter features the case of Elena and her family. I have chosen this case because it typifies the structural binds that characterize families' experiences of dealing with CKD and opens up a set of concerns that are traced outward in subsequent chapters. In the discussion that follows Elena's story, I draw particular attention to the labor families must engage in if they are to establish any coherence of care. Perpetual movement underpins this labor, as families like Elena's attempt to piece together a healthcare system for themselves. This movement is created out of radical contingency, the variability of fleeting encounters, and the windows of opportunity for treatment they present across only temporarily linkable sites, settings, and access regimes. I describe this as "government by movement" and use it to challenge the use of more standardized or ideal-typical accounts of biopolitical regimes. I argue that rather than being situated within an already definable apparatus of control—states, markets, medicine, welfare—that structures visible populations, the reverse is often the case. Rather than functioning as the *targets* of these domains, the practices of the mobile poor are *productive* of these domains.

Chapter 3, "Labor: Producing Sickness and the State," extends the previous discussion to advance understanding of the interface between labor, labor-market position, and health. Labor-market position, as in many other countries, is the key determinant of access to social insurance in Mexico and so determines social protection. In an increasingly flexibilized labor market, citizens move through various forms of work with the same precarity they do various forms of healthcare. Health insurance is lost regularly through redundancy, or gained in circumstances when patients come to informal arrangements with local employers. At times, families abandon their health insurance in the face of bottlenecks in the system, long waits, or dissatisfaction with services, choosing instead out-of-pocket expenses.

I draw on existing scholarship focusing on the state, welfare regimes, and worlds of work, labor, and citizenship to provide a detailed understanding of the emergence of Mexico's hybrid corporatist/neoliberal welfare state. As I will show, recent historical processes have culminated in a situation where Mexico's poor are increasingly locked out of social security entitlements and reliant on new private markets in healthcare, a development seen across countries well beyond Mexico today. By drawing on ethnographic data and interviews with patients, their families, Mexican scholars, and key actors in new healthcare industries, I discuss how patterns of inequality have emerged as a product of particular forms of welfare, highlighting what happens when access to healthcare is mediated through the cash nexus and a limited social rights agenda.

Next, chapter 4, "Brokering Healthcare: Paper-work, Negotiation, and the Strategies of Navigation," examines the local and particular interface between patient and doctor and the ways in which care for CKD and access to renal replacement therapies and drug treatments are negotiated. Drawing on observations and interviews within the context of clinical consultations, with reference to recent anthropological work on the cultural life of the bureaucratic document (Hull 2012a, 2012b), I explore the kinds of texts (scripts, prescriptions, letters of support, and more) produced within these clinical encounters, and the multiple readings and forms of interpretation they are open to. These highly contingent and unstable cultural objects, I argue, are not simply read but also acted on, in ways that are rarely easy to predict in advance.

Patients, for example, petition doctors to produce *resumés* for them. These are legitimating scripts, which patients must have when attempting to access support and broker healthcare across public, private, and charitable domains. Within the clinical encounter, doctors manipulate prescriptions for medications to increase access for the uninsured or increase prescription quantities so that those with access to forms of insurance can share with those without. These local and contingent arrangements underpin the vulnerability of care for patients, but also show doctors' practices to be highly circumscribed, despite their capacity to control the interfaces the poor must navigate. As a result, we see institutional actors, such as doctors, emerge as ambivalent agents of the state and market, who simultaneously embody and subvert their operations in the course of their everyday work.

The unpredictable lines of movement Mexican patients must take to secure support, as described in chapter 2, and the systemic and institutional arrangements that necessitate that movement, as discussed in chapters 3 and 4, mean that poor and sick bodies draw around them all manner of events, processes, and interactions that embody radically different kinds of exchange between very different kinds of actor. In taking up the idea that illness establishes transactions of many different kinds, chapter 5, "Exchange: Bodies as Sites for the Production of (Surplus) Value," draws on the well-established literature on exchange in anthropology, in particular how writings on the processes of gift-giving, commodification, and forms of reciprocity link together the social and the biological across both local and global terrains.

Rather than simply focusing attention on organs as the sole subject of exchange, my purpose here is to broaden our thinking to include the forms of exchange necessary for organ transplantation to occur. These include gifts solicited and unsolicited; conditional and unconditional forms of support; social transfers in the forms of benefits and social insurance payouts; contractual obligations, barter, and monetary exchange. These forms of exchange are organized around and (temporarily) stabilized by an unpredictably varied cast of agents, including kinship and friendship networks, charitable associations, and civil society organizations. These forms of exchange and the infrastructures of care they connect to are complex and contingent; they cannot be specified in advance. In this chapter, I argue that those at the periphery of social welfare and entitlement in Mexico have little choice but to link these modes of exchange together, in order to make healthcare work for them. In so doing, they co-produce new markets in medicine. Sick and poor bodies, as exhibited by a condition like CKD, are shown to be key sites in the production of surplus value and generative of the markets that transplant medicine increasingly depends on, a "vampiric" relation I discuss with reference to Marx.

Those relations are revealed in other ways, too. In 2008, Hospital Civil was embroiled in a major corruption and high-profile organ exchange scandal. The hospital had attracted one of the country's top surgeons, who had trained at the U.S. Mayo Clinic. He had almost singlehandedly accelerated the pace and rate of the transplant program during his time. He was found to be accepting large payments for transplanting the organs of wealthy patients who were not on the national waiting lists, amid rumors of organ trafficking, and was forced to leave in 2009. The event culminated in a massive rupture between the living organ and cadaveric transplant programs and their teams, and a massive political divide between university, medical, and city leaders. In chapter 6, "Transplant Scandals, the State, and the 'Multiple Problematics' of Accountability," I examine the different reports of this event, drawing on them to (re)think the ways in which scandals and incidences of malpractice or malfeasance have structured accounts of transplant medicine across anthropological literatures; I show, too, how they provide an important guide to understanding the role of governance and power as they are bound up with the lucrative growth of technoscientific interventions. The key objective of this chapter is to question how scandals serve to draw a boundary between the "good" and the "bad," the "benign" and the "malignant" within transplant medicine. Scandals serve to render locally organized forms of transplant medicine *ordinary*, even when those *ordinary* ways of working can be seen, when approached slightly differently, as anything but—particularly when viewed in terms of their catastrophic repercussions for individuals and their families.

Moving from the role of scandal in the diffusion of transplant medicine, in chapter 7, "Political and Corporate Etiologies: Producing Disease Emergence and Disease Response," I look at one of the emerging crises to which transplant medicine has been presented as a response. In Mexico today, the rise of CKD is not only associated with a rise in diabetes and hypertension but is also linked to instances of state and corporate harm by virtue of an unregulated food industry, poor toxic waste management, unchecked use of pesticides, impoverished working conditions, and environmental pollution. In Mexico, this is also seen as the legacy of NAFTA—the effect of trade agreements that have seen indigenous industry and labor rights suffer as multi- and transnational corporations enjoy an incentivized and deregulated market for their goods. The repercussions of these structures of production and consumption for the health of Mexico's citizens have barely begun to be calculated. The evidence needed to do so does not exist due to the absence of any systematic program for gathering epidemiological and toxicological data. Among other things, Mexico also lacks an effective apparatus of counting and population surveillance. It does not have a nationally organized kidney registry, nor an integrated epidemiology of kidney disease. While the scale and burden of chronic conditions like CKD have generated intense debate about challenges for prevention and monitoring, CKD currently inhabits an epistemological shadow zone. This raises very interesting questions about the stability of a more familiar biopolitical apparatus, of the kind we might assume is at play in Anglo-American contexts.

In working this idea through, I draw attention to the varied processes of knowledge production as well as the corporate and political etiologies that shape the processes of disease emergence and organize responses to it. Both problem and solution—CKD and transplant medicine—are shown to be formed out of the same basic stuff. The articulation of one is essentially the articulation of the other. Although this relationship is explicated in context-sensitive terms, with attention to the place of sickness and healthcare in Mexico's neoconservative economy, valuable lessons are drawn from the Mexican case that have relevance for an understanding of the political economy at the heart of a much broader global health agenda.

1 · STUDYING REGIMES OF RENAL CARE

The challenges faced by the patients we met in the introductory chapter—Alicia, Carlos, Luis, and Julio, and their respective families—offer a distinct vantage point onto regimes of renal care, one occupied from positions barely maintained at the margins of welfare and entitlement. The particularities of an individual's encounters with those regimes open up Mexico's multi-tiered healthcare system for scrutiny, exposing who has access to what, when, and via which means. Through the work they have to do to secure and retain access, Mexico's uninsured pull into view alternative modes of navigating, accessing, resourcing, producing, and consuming healthcare to show that life on the margins is far from a marginal concern but is, instead, of central importance.

In this chapter, I turn to the regimes of renal care at work in Mexico; those revealed in painful patient journeys, which include the organ replacement technologies of transplantation and dialysis, but also extend beyond them. I use the term *regimes* to indicate that these forms of treatment and intervention are neither fixed nor universal, but have, instead, stabilized over time as culturally and institutionally recognized ways of organizing treatment and care. This usage is an explicit borrowing from the writing of the *regulation school*, with its origins in 1970s French political economy and its emphasis on the ways in which systems of capital accumulation become regularized over time, expressing the various social relations (economic and non-economic) of production, consumption, circulation, and so on (Boyer 1990).[1] Systems of healthcare are no less contingent on these social relations and, thus, the notion of regimes of renal care is useful as it directs our attention outward to the ways in which the provision of healthcare is fundamentally tied to a political economy.

Nevertheless, any discussion of renal care regimes poses a series of more specific questions: what exactly are they? Where do we find them? How do they work? Do their features change from place to place? One of the core recommendations of this book is that there is no invariable core to these renal care regimes those questions can be meaningfully asked of. Instead, through an engagement with the particularities of specific cases, via ongoing, often localized processes of interpretation, adaptation, and (re)configuration, we come to understand the global spread of renal care. As the chapters of this book show, we arrive at a better understanding of the general based on our encounters with the specifics. Indeed, renal care regimes, typically organized with organ transplantation and forms of dialysis at their center, are continuously being elaborated and built upon out of the specifics. In recognizing this, we see that the Mexican case helps us arrive at answers to the questions listed above in two ways: first, it shows, ontologically and substantively, *what* precisely we are faced with when we encounter regimes of renal care, while methodologically it shows us *how* to study their arrangements and *which* resources we need to do so.

So first, *what* is it we are faced with? What might we take regimes of renal care in Mexico to be? How we tackle the specifics of what we set out to study is a recurring question for anthropologists and sociologists and emerges every time we are faced with macro forms of organization: society, the state, healthcare, and so on. Reflecting on that question, Callon and Latour (1981) trouble the very nature of the "what" in their reworking of Hobbes's account of the state—the body of Leviathan. In trying to understand Leviathan, they suggest, we are presented with a cacophony of "monstrous" metaphors: of bodies; of machines; of systems of exchange; of physical interactions. They say:

> One can never describe the whole set of elements using only one set of these metaphors . . . we [are always forced to] jump from one . . . to another . . . Monstrous [indeed] is the Leviathan [therefore] . . . This is because . . . there is not just one Leviathan but many, interlocked one into another like chimera, each one claiming to represent the reality of all, the programme of the whole. (Callon and Latour 1981, 294)

What we might take from Callon and Latour is that we cannot analyze renal regimes, just as we cannot analyze Leviathan, if we treat them as fixed and unitary or try to make one of their interlocked constituents "represent the reality of all." Leviathan isn't an undifferentiated whole and neither are regimes of renal care. They do not have well-defined boundaries, nor are they sealed off from the world but, instead, leak outward into it. As a consequence, it is difficult to immediately see the arrangements particular regimes depend on and that serve to fasten them in place.

This applies as much to seemingly more stable aspects of renal care—like transplant medicine—as its less stable, more obviously socially, culturally, and economically variable features. As I was reminded on my first day of fieldwork, transplant and renal care programs, in the UK, for example, would not begin, as they do in Mexico, without resources. The understood and felt dysfunctions of transplant medicine and renal care in Mexico elicited reflection on what doctors often assumed were smoother processes and operations in other parts of the world. National comparisons had the effect of seeming to make invisible elsewhere what was dramatically and continually in relief for Mexican medical staff: an exclusionary and stratified political economy of healthcare, one encountered here as the lack of provision; falling levels of medically trained personnel; inadequate numbers of hospital beds; poor medical equipment; insufficient varieties of drugs or stocks of blood; weak administrative infrastructures; poorly coordinated strategies for health promotion and health education, and many other things. The articulation of institutional shortcomings in Mexico also had the effect of assuming that transplant medicine, and the regimes of care into which it was woven, could in more "developed" contexts *comparatively* be taken for granted, made to recede into the background by its general friction-free functioning and stable, predictable organization. Renal care and transplant medicine in the UK were assumed to function in such a way that they broadly fitted to demand, resources, and general service expectations, and although that is an over-simplification, within limits, there may be some truth to it. However, whatever the accuracy of the comparison, the point the doctors were making was that in Mexico, in the public health system, the infrastructure of transplantation and renal care could never be taken for granted. In tracing its operations, I came to see this too. Wherever I looked, I was continually confronted with a profoundly discordant and disruptive set of interventions at play, ones that inhabited and often capitalized on the precarious interface between human suffering and resource allocation.

Given transplantation's iconic status and position at the apex of renal care, it is a useful place to start to trace these issues further. Comparative and cross-cultural research in anthropology has shown that organ transplantation is not a discrete technology—that is, something that simply facilitates the moving of one kidney into the body of another (Cohen 2002; Crowley-Matoka 2005; Hamdy 2010; Kierans 2015; Lock 2001; Manderson 2011; Scheper-Hughes 2008). It is, instead, part of a wider apparatus of techniques, knowledge, and resources constructed piecemeal in particular contexts (Ingold 2000). No country ever develops a fully operational transplant medicine program from a standing start; it has to be slowly assembled. If we are to give proper consideration to what makes the biomedical and technological interventions bound up with this aspect of renal care appropriate or inappropriate, then, we have to learn how that process works and what its implications are, how it is indigenized and put to work, what constitutes its specific role in healthcare in terms of alleviating or creating human suffering, and, in the end, who benefits.

At the same time, while organ transplant programs are assembled and adapted for local use, developing and thus changing over time, they have to have some stable elements. There has to be some consensus as to what they are and do and why, indeed, they are needed at all. They have to stand, somehow, by the facts and claims that are produced about them, such as the accepted premise that kidney transplantation is a fixed human good driven by a moral imperative to save life and the optimum treatment for chronic kidney disease (CKD). However, if we start off by characterizing kidney transplantation in this way, we are likely to take its consequences for granted as well as the deep political work of making the technology in the first place. Its actual functioning would become a residual category, something that would only show up when we examine why things don't work as they should. We would confuse (claims about) what transplant medicine "ought" to be with what it actually "is." The tactic I adopt, informed by this, is not to subordinate the "is" to the "ought," sublimating the living worlds of transplant technology to an abstract moral vision, but to suspend an interest in "the ought" in order to better understand, in adapting Marx (1970 [1844]), "actually existing" organ transplantation and its place within practices of renal care. We cannot understand renal care without understanding organ transplantation. It is central to it as the promise people, whose efforts are invested into attaining a new organ, are sold. It is assumed as an end point (Kierans 2005). Organ transplantation, however, is but one of several technological anchor points used to secure renal care, which include different modalities of dialysis and pharmaceutical interventions, among others (Manderson 2011).

To understand "actually existing" forms of organ transplantation and to see the deep political work of making the technologies of renal care in the first place, Shapin and Schaffer (1985) offer a place to begin. Taking Robert Boyle's air pump as an exemplar, they show how it acquired stability as a fact, as a particular thing in the world. They contend that the success of the air pump simultaneously rested on what they refer to as three constitutive "technologies": (a) a material technology, one embodied in the construction, operation, and material integrity of the apparatus; (b) a literary technology, a means by which the phenomena produced by the apparatus could be made known to those who were not direct witnesses; and (c) a social technology that incorporated the conventions—the rules of conduct—experimental philosophers should abide by in dealing with each other in considering, evaluating, and reproducing knowledge claims.

Of course, unlike Boyle's experimental set ups, we cannot assign a physical integrity to the technologies of organ replacement or definitively fix their boundaries. We can, however, trace the genealogies of the components from which they have been assembled over time. Lawrence Cohen (2004, 168–169), for instance, shows us that organ transplantation and associated technologies of care were dependent on three broad technical shifts across the twentieth century. According to Cohen, these were (1) the development of mechanical techniques for safely and effectively extracting, transporting, and grafting tissues, based on the outcome of the work of surgical pioneers such as Alexis Carrel, awarded the Nobel Prize in 1912 for establishing vascular suturing techniques; (2) the development of immunological techniques—themselves an outcome of transfusion medicine during two world wars—which showed how tissue rejection could be minimized, and in so doing, facilitated the demarcations of "bioavailability" by identifying who could serve as organ donors; and (3) the (fortuitous) identification, development, and manufacture of immunosuppressant drugs, in particular cyclosporine, discovered by chance in moss while bio-prospecting in Scandinavian fjords. This has helped curb the perennial problem of organ rejection and has contributed to the globalization of organ donation, and it has also established the need for new regimes of pre- and post-transplant care, patient preparation, and so on.

These developments owe much to successive and prior innovations in knowledge, technique, and practice, such as advances in blood transfusion, pioneered in the early 1800s, and skin grafting techniques, developed some decades later. It was not, however, until Peter Medawar identified the immunological processes that underlay tissue rejection, thereby establishing the principles of histocompatibility, that the mechanics of organ transplantation were established.

Further to these developments is the central provision of life-support by the respiratory ventilator and the increasing sophistication of intensive-care medicine and its associated technologies: the electrocardiogram and the techniques of defibrillation. Over 400 different ventilators have been developed since the first: the artificial lung in the mid-nineteenth century (Lock 2001). Ventilation ensures that the body's organs remain oxygenated and so preserved in an optimum state for transplantation. It has served, in turn, to produce the category of brain-death and a new ontological entity: the "living cadaver" (Lock 1995, 2001; Sharp 2006). The modalities of dialysis (hemodialysis and peritoneal) also have their roots in mid-nineteenth-century discoveries and breakthroughs. They have been critical to the transplant project, to stabilizing patients with CKD, by filtering toxins from the bloodstream, thereby sustaining bodily functioning while patients wait for a kidney. Dialysis, in other words, widens the pool of potential organ recipients that transplant medicine can render its services to.

No technology, however, is simply the sum of its infrastructures. How the complex of transplant technology has been taken up, practiced, and accepted is, in Shapin and Schaffer's terms, also a "literary" concern, one of immense sociological and anthropological importance. The various modes of storytelling and narrative work that drive organ replacement and exchange have been shown to be fundamental to its stabilization and public acceptance, to how it "has taken root with little opposition" (Lock 1995, 391). Attending to these literary/discursive forms lays bare the assumptions underpinning organ transplantation, unfolding its ideology. Lesley Sharp distils these as an amalgam of paradoxical devices that incorporate:

(1) the concept of transplantation as a medical miracle; (2) the denial of transplantation as a form of body commodification; (3) the perception of transplantable organs as precious things; (4) the dependence on brain death criteria for generating

transplantable parts; (5) the assertion that organs of human origin are becoming increasingly scarce in our society and require radical solutions; (6) an insistence that the melding of disparate bodies is part of a natural progression in a medical realm predicated on technological expertise; and, finally, (7) the imperative that compassion and trust remain central to the care of dying patients, even when a new corporate style of medicine demands an increasing number of transplantable organs. (2006, 8)

Sharp opens up the contours of this literary technology, revealing richly textured forms of storytelling, assertive in their construction and persuasive in their force. They are, furthermore, organized around a set of key tropes: the idea that organ transplantation is the optimal (cost-effective) solution, particularly given escalations in CKD the world over; a politics of scarcity that continues to fuel innovation in transplant medicine and the demand for donated organs, among many other forms of exchange and transfer; the gift of life metaphor that has fostered organ donation as an acceptable practice in many parts of the world; and the heroism of a pioneering profession, which ensures that organ transplantation continues to be seen as one of the great miracles of modern science.

Just as no technology is the sum of its infrastructures, it cannot be reduced to its justificatory narratives either. Taken alone, these are incomplete. Put simply, people are required. They are implicated in the transplant project and the systems organ transplantation has found a place within, in various ways. For one thing, people are needed to advance those justificatory narratives in the appropriate times and places and to tailor those material technologies and infrastructures for use in particular contexts. Transplant medicine is a practical concern, the work of many hands, and that work must somehow be organized and coordinated if it is to function. Ways have to be found of connecting people together for specific tasks and to anchor their efforts to the wider enterprise. In establishing the practical ground of organ transplantation, a range of potent "social technologies" thus have to be developed and brought into play in various different places.

Social technologies are diffuse, and therefore difficult to pin down across various national and international domains. The following practices, however, might be said to characterize social relations in this domain: *practices of inscription*, such as instructional/directive writing, and the pragmatic literatures they produce (research reports, academic papers, policy documents, regulations, codes of practice, protocols, patient files); *dissemination fora* (conferences, workshops, teaching fora, symposia); and *associational networks* (built up through practitioner connections, hierarchies and statuses, professional associations, extra-medical associations [market and governmental links], various patient bodies, forms of charity and patronage). These are all underpinned by distinct discursive repertories (disciplinary and professional languages: written, statistical, and representational). In sum, social technologies provide a means of demarcating, delineating, and giving shape to those collective practices that consolidate a technological apparatus and the regimes of care it is connected to over time through the hands-on work of communities of practitioners and other relevant parties (like patients). Different from the work of a literary technology, these are the contexts within which medical knowledge comes to be established rather than justified, shown rather than told, where the facts of the matter not only acquire stability, but do so in terms of the forms of language, rhetoric, and representation through which their stability is displayed.

In Mexico, these practitioner communities are characterized by organizations such as the Mexican Transplant Society, The Mexican College of Nephrologists, The Mexican Institute of Nephrology Research, the National Association of Nephrology of Mexico, and the National Council of Nephrology, as well as those charged with the promotion, governance, and wider organization of organ transplantation. All are affiliated to and participate in wider international networks, although it could be argued that, as representatives of various national medical interests, not everyone participates on equal terms. By way of example, the World Congress of Nephrology is a bi-annual event established by the International Society of Nephrology. Its goal is the worldwide advancement of education, science and patient care; it constitutes an international platform for scientific exchange and to address disparities in the access and resourcing of renal and transplant medicine. However, efforts to address concerns around global health inequalities has led to the formation of an affiliated satellite symposium held after the main event, with the sole intention of discussing kidney disease among so called "disadvantaged" populations and so reflecting the challenges of addressing health in low- and middle-income countries. Its satellite status, however, is double-edged. On the one hand, it has become necessary to separate the subject of resourcing and access to transplant medicine from scientific and technical issues, for fear of being subsumed by them; but this separation also creates a marginality of concern. Establishing an appropriate platform for the wide range of issues that underpin the practice and growth of organ transplantation is a perennial source of tension between the various organizing committees and geographic interests. In addition, what gets to be discussed and with what discursive tools—numeric/clinical lab results, epidemiological statistics, descriptive social science accounts—reflects the different social, cultural, and political values attached to various theoretical and technical responses to the problems of health and technology in different places.

Shapin and Schaffer's technologies—material, literary, and social—help us to avoid taking the contemporary technologies of renal care for granted as fixed human goods, from assuming its consequences in advance or from black-boxing its operations. Beyond the properties of these interlinked technologies, the differentiated apparatuses that enable the transfer of organs from one body to another and the modes of exchange they depend on ensure that regimes of renal care take different forms and follow different trajectories—social, cultural, political, economic, and moral—in different places. Shapin and Schaffer's technologies are a useful analytical starting point for describing these regimes, but they do not tell us how or where to proceed, or how to acquire an understanding of their forms and functions from one site to another.

By virtue of the processes in and through which renal care finds a place in different contexts, it has reach and extension. Once a particular regime takes root, it reconfigures the socio-political environment it inhabits, shaping and being shaped in equal measure through the kinds of feedback loops Ian Hacking (1995) suggests are features of onto-genesis—the practical making and remaking of human worlds. To understand regimes of renal care, from transplantation through dialysis to screening and monitoring practices, we must therefore treat what would count as understanding as an empirical concern, first and foremost. This means we have to see *how* they work in practice. To do this, as this book shows, we have to start somewhere.

EMBARKING ON PATIENT JOURNEYS

So, how do we proceed? I start with those seeking out renal care—patients, their families, and the journeys they have to take to secure care for CKD in the context of the specific regimes that care is structured around. These are the patients whose kidneys have failed; the majority of them young, poor, and living outside Mexico's systems of entitlements to healthcare. All are in need of or have already acquired an organ transplant; most are dependent on their families to provide these much-needed organs as well as the much-needed moral and material resources to make an organ transplant possible.

Following them and their modes of engagement with organ replacement technologies takes us to the many sites within and across which renal care regimes are articulated and which are flexibly joined together by them: hospitals, clinics, home dialysis settings, charitable organizations, pharmaceutical companies, pharmacies, social work departments, and the city streets of Guadalajara. These routes to care introduce us to the range of social actors who inhabit, populate, and are variously enrolled into renal regimes, whose alliances make its operations possible: doctors, nurses, policy makers, money lenders, black market medication sellers, journalists, researchers, government officials, bureaucrats, among others. This is in addition to the multitude of paperwork, objects, and equipment that stabilize and facilitate its operations: transplant protocols, medication prescriptions, resumés, x-rays, exam results, catheters, biopsy needles, dialysis machines, newspaper articles, trade agreements, and so on. Taken together—though far from comprehensive or final—these heterogeneous elements show up the "obligatory points of passage" (Callon 1986) that constitute and animate renal care, while marking out the biopolitical terrain that characterizes it. This complex of arrangements is not simply a reflection of its environment but worked into it. It grows and spreads by virtue of its reflexive adaptation to local conditions. By harnessing the possibilities of those local conditions, it is made to function. This is what gives renal care its specificity and character, but it is also what shows us why there are no clear points of contrast to compare across settings. To understand them, we must explore them in situ.

The lives and journeys of Mexican patients and their families tell multiple stories—stories of profound suffering and sacrifice are certainly prominent among them. However, this book is not about the patient experience per se and the analyses I offer are not just there to persuade the reader of the suffering of those whose situations I have set out. Instead, I ask what these experiences and sufferings point outward to; what they can teach us about this complex regime; how it is made to work; the system of alliances it depends on; the political economy it is grounded in; the biopolitics it gives rise to, and, indeed, the work of the state conducted through and by it. The lives of these patients demonstrate the importance of seeing activity at the intersections and associations between macro and micro forces as sites where regimes of care are made and re-made pragmatically by those implicated in them. This means as ethnographers—as Callon and Latour (1981) suggest—we follow these associations and disassociations as they are produced. Said another way, it is not simply the patients and their families who are put on the move by seeking out regimes of renal care; so, too is the anthropologist in the course of her work.

PUTTING THE ANALYST ON THE MOVE

In tracing the journeys patients and their families take, we will be brought, in the chapters that follow, directly to Mexico's systems of welfare and from there to the systematic state failures embodied within a fragmented and deliberately segmented welfare state. Understanding the role and functions of the welfare state in the context of renal care is not, however, wholly self-evident from the outset. With Max Weber's comments about the rational-legal character of bureaucracy somewhere perhaps in the back of our minds, we might expect that the structure of welfare arrangements should tell us who has access to what, and relatively unambiguously so. However, that turns out to be misconceived. Instead, ambiguity and fluidity of status turns out to be the rule and not the exception. Patients' journeys thus point us "onward" to the political economy of the welfare state but only to then take us back to patients' journeys again, revealing another aspect of their centrality. While the organization of welfare and entitlement is of course important (see chapters 2 and 3 for a description), it is only by returning to the people themselves and the labor they engage in that we learn about the particular functions and dysfunctions of the welfare state for those who must work to make up for its limitations and neglectful dispassion or side-step its inefficiencies. Again, we have to start with the patient, not a formal description of government or the welfare state, if we are to fully understand the space the Mexican renal regime actually occupies. When we do, we come to see it is indeed, in part, a bureaucratic space, but not as that is ordinarily imagined.

Nor do patient journeys unfold in isolation. The labor of patients and their families is inevitably mediated, regularly and routinely undertaken at the interface between them and their doctors, through the production and accumulation of paper-work (see chapter 4). Paper-work, such as hospital files, x-rays, exam results, prescriptions, and so on, accompany patients on their journeys toward care. Paper-work grounds encounters, while facilitating and furthering others. Paper-work keeps things moving. It materializes the condition, but it does not formalize or fix it. It does not produce a formal record of it, it does not give the CKD patient a resting point, nor does it legitimize the labor of the patient. In keeping patients on the move, paper-work responsibilizes them as the principal agent for the treatment of their condition.

Being on the move is, thus, critical, pragmatically and analytically. Indeed, the population of uninsured, unentitled patients is constituted by virtue of the requirement to move in the first place. Movement affords this population visibility in the absence of integrated state systems of data sharing between hospitals or organized kidney registries. It shows that these patients are not situated within an already definable apparatus of control or surveillance by the state as one might expect from standard accounts of biopolitical regimes. Rather, that very apparatus of control—the work of the state—is itself made tangible and real by virtue of their movements. The wider political economic conditions within which regimes of renal care take root, that link together systems of welfare, the market, and medicine are thus yet another site of state-making. It is this we as analysts are taken to. It is here we see its work modulated and exercised and where we see the profound dispossessions and harms that occur when the state fails to ensure adequate compensation, entitlement, and protections to its citizens, leaving them to the mercy of new markets and forms of exchange that have insinuated themselves in Mexican healthcare. They too are pulled into view by the movement of patients. The renal care regime, as a consequence, overspills, spreading out into the wider culture, society, political system, and economy. As a consequence, cultural, social, political, and economic practices come to be reconfigured so that people can respond to, invest in, or capitalize on that overspill.

It is within these highly contingent circumstances that renal care can produce arbitrary outcomes, leading to harm, sickness, organ rejection, dispossession, catastrophic impoverishment, death—where the labor of the patient and their families is emptied out to the point of depletion. These harms, as I will point out throughout the book, are unexceptional. They are a taken-for-granted feature of contemporary Mexican life. They are ordinary state failures, made possible by a social production of indifference (Herzfeld 1992), despite the best efforts of all those involved to provide a care that can never quite materialize as such. These mundane and routine state failures are dramatically thrown into relief when things go drastically wrong, in the case of medical malpractice and the abuse of office. In these instances, the entire apparatus of transplant medicine can be short-circuited. Here not only are the state and its obligations further pulled into view, so is the entire system of governance that organizes, houses, and makes possible renal care as actually practiced: its institutional ground.

ORGANS AS ANCHORS

In considering the location of renal care regimes, one feature that holds across sites and situations is that they are fixed to the fact of a failing organ; fixed to the fact of CKD as the material ground of sickness. It is through CKD that they gain purchase—CKD is its raison d'être. CKD is on the rise in Mexico, as is the unruly, unexplained variant of it, CKDu. As CKD spreads, so too does the renal regime. It insinuates itself with the condition that provides not only the ground for its extensions but also the possibilities and limits of the regime itself. Here problem and solution, cause and care, mirror each other in locally defined and meaning-ful ways. Both extend from the same social, economic, and political conditions. CKDu, however, is of particular concern, as it changes the terms upon which trans-plant medicine and renal care justify and articulate themselves. In many respects, CKDu dismantles the mythology of organ transplantation, particularly that which extends from living-related donors, the predominant mode of transfer in Mexico. Lesley Sharp (2006) reminds us that living organ donation assumes no harm to a healthy donor, that the remaining, other, kidney provides the necessary func-tions needed to maintain a healthy body. This is a justification of its practice. This assumption, however, is increasingly difficult to maintain in all contexts, but par-ticularly so in countries where CKD extends itself as an outcome of poverty, pre-carity, and degraded environments and where kidneys are offered by those who are already vulnerable and cannot be said to be healthy donors. In the course of fieldwork, I have heard on more than one occasion a diagnosis of CKD given to an organ donor, threatening the viability of their remaining, other "healthy" kid-ney. This calls into question the stories we can tell about the merits and possibili-ties of transplant medicine and renal care. Setting out in clearer ways the terms of "the gift" being offered sharpens the endpoints and sets the boundaries to the transplant project and regimes of renal care, while demonstrating more perspic-uously how they fix themselves to the failing organ.

What, then, are the prospects for renal care? This is a question continually raised by the ethnographic accounts that follow. In a context of poverty, profound social inequality, systemic welfare fragmentation, and encroaching private mar-kets in healthcare, can actually existing renal regimes be said to provide a way of caring, when they, themselves, by virtue of their restricted modes of access, are implicated in the exacerbation of inequality, destructive of the moral economy of family and community, and harmful to the people they seek to help? The pressures on these resource-intensive technologies of care are only set to worsen as the demographic groups who must rely on them get younger and the diagnostic tools used alongside them prove incapable of coping with the rise and spread of failing organs. If elements of this set of arrangements are not revisited and changed, renal care will become bound up with the destruction of life, rather than the stabilization or saving of life.

Hannah Arendt's reflection on the conditions of possibility for "future man" is one that resonates with transplant medicine, renal care, and their prospects. Much like the transplant recipient or the dialysis patient whose embodied status relies on the bodies of others or the assistance of machines, Arendt's "future man" is also a hybrid being, one with the potential to embody both the lived relations of domination and possibility. Arendt sees this hybrid being as made by science and possessed "by a rebellion against human existence as it has been given, a free gift from nowhere (secularly speaking)" (1998 [1958], 2–3). She contends that there is no reason to doubt our abilities to create new living forms, just as there is no reason to doubt our ability to destroy organic life. She questions only whether we wish to use our scientific and technical knowledge for these ends. Arendt (1998 [1958]) understands that the question she is posing is inherently political; however, it is one that cannot be decided by professional scientists, nor professional politicians. Renal care regimes as they extend into various global sites and settings take up her question. They make visible the conditions of possibility for Arendt's "future man" and, as the chapters that follow show, it is in doing so that they have, and make, politics.

Renal care regimes are deeply and contextually reflexive. They are not epiphenomena, not merely products of an environment, but have lives of their own, ones that extend by virtue of their technological affordances. To function, specific regimes rely on alliances between medicine, the market, and the state but are themselves involved in establishing those alliances. These are not the same in all places and they are not visible from above, nor from outside their systems of functioning. They are only visible from within, from the vantage points supplied by the practices of those whose efforts are required to keep the regime in place, and which, in turn, make visible its particular form and articulations.

Renal care can and does, however, appear as if it is solid, a thing in and of the world, a set of discernible actions and practices. Underpinning the production of its appearances, interrogating its matter-of-factness reveals tangled and often troubling fields of action and technological practice, which, in the context of this book, comprise the objects of methodological attention—renal care itself. In the chapters that follow, I do not intend to map out or produce a comprehensive description of such practices but, rather, document and identify what precisely shows up in the context of Mexico's living-organ donor program, to show how these "matters-of-fact" are transformed into particular matters-of-concern in Mexico and beyond (Latour 2004; Lynch 2008). Shapin and Schaffer's three "technologies" (1985) serve both as analytical resources and sensitizing devices to do just that. They help us to understand that the conditions within which transplant and renal care technologies take root—those supplied by the operations of nation states, markets, regimes of government—do not come pre-formed. I am, therefore, interested in what Michael Lynch, following Alfred Schutz and Harold Garfinkel, calls the topic/resource distinction; in this case, the practices and conditions of possibility that enable us to see the technologies of transplant medicine come as part of the everyday lives of individuals. These conditions of possibility become analytical circumstances of relevance for the chapters that follow (Lynch 2008).

2 · BIOPOLITICS AND THE ANALYTICS OF A POPULATION ON THE MOVE

Transplant medicine is not only one of the most technologized domains of scientific medicine; it is also one of the most globalized, with kidney transplants now carried out in over ninety-one countries (Shimazono 2007). This is significant, given the steady rise of CKD worldwide, making it one of the fastest-rising causes of death today. Mexico is cited as having the highest CKD death-rate in the world (Lange Neuen et al. 2017), exemplifying CKD's disproportionate effects on those living in the global south—countries for whom the provision of and access to kidney transplantation are a perennial cause for concern.[1]

In Mexico, the desire to enhance the provision and extend the reach of transplant medicine is critical to strategies for managing the nation's kidney disease problem, but it is also important to the country's drive for modernization and development: an aspiration to distance itself from the effects of traditionalism and dependency. As Crowley-Matoka (2016) notes, this desire was articulated in the early 2000s, with the election of Vincente Fox and the defeat of PRI after seventy years in power.[2] Fox wanted to create a new place for Mexico in a globalized and globalizing world by building closer ties to the U.S. business community and breaking with the country's stagnant and corrupt past (Crowley-Matoka 2016). Organ transplantation was to be marshalled as part of this narrative of progress, helping to steer Mexico's final emergence into modernity. What would emerge in actuality was a medical system that continued to be deeply fractured by political economy, leading to the partial construction of a transplant infrastructure unable to meet the needs of the country's rising CKD population.

The challenge of developing a renal care infrastructure was a source of pre-occupation and frustration for medical staff working in the public hospital. There was much talk about the Mexican Ministry of Health's stated commitment to expanding the provision of renal replacement therapies—forms of dialysis and transplantation—to those without sufficient means, but promises to make the necessary resources available rarely moved beyond political overtures. Like the two doctors mentioned in the introduction, attempting to push through their cargo of dialysate solution into the nephrology ward, most healthcare professionals I spoke to about transplant medicine would point outward beyond the clinical arena to implicate state and federal administrations when assigning responsibility and blame; such pointing itself a distinctly political act. Each time I was party to such conversations, I was aware that, in assigning political accountability, what was being pointed out was generally something imagined to hover above or beyond an impoverished medical infrastructure from which the Mexican state was detached with the power to constrain or enable what medics wished to see happen. While the Mexican case has much to teach us about complex forms of power and the various mechanisms used in their exercise, I am interested in the particular ways in which such forms of power are revealed by those directly engaged in the work of medicine. And so, when protagonists attempt to show us where power lies, it is always important to ask what else is being done or said, and to think about what might be at stake in demarcating the boundaries of the political. Before moving on to these more analytical concerns, however, some additional scene-setting is needed. I therefore provide a brief description of Mexico's transplant project to show how the challenges it faces have come to be framed and understood.

The first kidney transplant in Mexico was carried out on 22 October 1963 at the Hospital General del Centro Médico Nacional (General Hospital of the National Medical Centre) of the Mexican Institute of Social Security (IMSS), a tertiary-level public hospital in Mexico City (Gracida-Juárez et al. 2011). As Treviño-Becerra (2007) recounts in his published reflection on the development of kidney care in Mexico, hemodialysis expanded alongside transplant medicine during the 1960s, but only as a bridging therapy for patients waiting for a transplant. Peritoneal dialysis, at this time, was in its infancy, administered in only two hospitals in Mexico City to patients with acute renal failure. Over the next two decades, he explains, both modalities expanded slowly, primarily in the hospitals of IMSS, due to close cooperation between medical staff and the country's main medical suppliers: Baxter, PiSA, and Fresenius. Efforts to establish peritoneal programs came under scrutiny and criticism as poor results and increasing costs necessitated greater scientific rigor and the monitoring of provision. Treviño-Becerra explains that as transplant waiting lists grew, patients petitioned the National Commission for Human Rights, as well as various medical organizations— many taking legal action—to be included in the small number of hemodialysis programs that were available. Despite this, by 1993, 93 percent of patients receiving dialysis therapy in Mexico were relying on peritoneal dialysis. In the following years, submissions were made to federal government by COMPETIRC (a national committee established for the treatment of CKD) to increase financial support for dialysis provision and to recalibrate the ratios of use between peritoneal and hemodialysis to 60:40 respectively, a re-balancing of targets that has yet to be met.[3] Peritoneal dialysis remains the country's modality of choice, due to its comparatively low cost for the state. Conventionally carried out in the patient's home and requiring the training of nominated caregivers as well as documented assurances that the appropriate conditions for its use are adhered to (Padilla-Altamira 2017), peritoneal dialysis incurs great personal costs, on an open-ended basis, for those families who have little choice but to accommodate it within the context of their home and family life, as I discuss in chapter 3.

The development of kidney transplantation and its associated replacement therapies is difficult to capture in straightforward or linear terms. It is particularly difficult to trace developments in medical care given the disunified character of Mexican health services. Kidney transplantation, like peritoneal dialysis, has evolved in ways that put the family front and center. In transplantation, that is, the family has become the principal source of the materials upon which this technology depends. In Jalisco, data gathered from the IMSS-affiliated Western Medical Centre suggests that for the period 1994–2014, 89 percent of organs were donated from living donors, with only 13 percent of these genetically unrelated (Solis-Vargas, Evangelista-Carrillo, and Puetes-Camacho 2016). This places organ donation firmly within the domain of kinship, a domain that is saturated by social relations and cultural expectations (Crowley-Matoka 2016). According to the WHO Global Observatory on Donation and Transplantation, Mexico carries out the fourth-highest number of living-donor transplants after the United States, India, and Turkey (White et al. 2014), a ranking that, when placed in context, is not quite the accomplishment it might first appear to be.

For countries who are dependent on this mode of transfer, we can expect to encounter differences in the ways transplant medicine has been accommodated and institutionalized in those settings—settings often characterized by non-universal healthcare systems with high relative up-front expenses. This is certainly the case in Mexico. Access to and organization of transplant services—as with all health services in Mexico—is fragmented, characterized by profound inequalities and administered by way of a complex quasi-insurance-based social security system linked to labor market position (Garcia-Diaz and Sosa-Rubi 2011; Frenk et al. 2006). Under this system, private-sector salaried workers and their families are covered by the Instituto Mexicano de Seguro Social (IMSS, the Mexican Institute of Social Security). The IMSS covers approximately 44 percent of the population, and 82 percent of those with health insurance, making it Mexico's largest healthcare provider. Beyond IMSS, the Instituto de Seguridad y Servicios Sociales de los Trabajadores de Estado (ISSSTE, the Institute of Social Security and Services for Civil Servants) provides services for federal workers and civil servants, accounting for approximately 5 percent of the population. Smaller social insurance systems also exist for those working in nationalized industries such as PEMEX (Mexican Petroleum). Private health insurers for highly paid workers constitute about 2 percent of the whole (INEGI 2011). For those not covered by any insurance—almost half the population, mainly informal, flexible workers, and the unemployed—services are generally provided at a subsidized cost by the clinics and hospitals of the Secretaria de Salud (the Ministry of Health). This safety net is run with no premiums, no guaranteed package of services, and at a significant cost to those who use it. Services are limited, often unavailable, and heavily reliant on out-of-pocket payments at the point of use.

Each of these systems provides its own idiosyncratic route through primary, secondary, and tertiary services and, in turn, access to renal replacement therapies. However, regardless of the seemingly fixed formal divisions around which provision is organized, distinctions between healthcare systems should be seen as fluid, with the regular movement of patients between them. Despite class or income levels, patients attempt, as personal means and opportunity allow, to make up for systemic limitations—such as the bottlenecks and long waits that have become associated with care in IMSS—by forgoing their social insurance entitlements to pay out of pocket in private clinics or at the services of the Ministry of Health and Welfare. As Crowley-Matoka (2016, 20) explains:

> Nationally, IMSS possessed the best developed infrastructure of clinics, hospitals, and specialized equipment of any of the Mexican health-care institutions—including the private sector. Yet IMSS clinics and hospitals were typically overburdened and undersupplied, and many patients who had rights to the system often opted for private care for minor ailments when they could afford it, in order to avoid long waits, out-of-stock pharmacies, and care that could be notoriously brusque. Deeply flawed but also deeply necessary as the primary source of health care for the majority of Mexicans, IMSS was regarded by many as one of the last remnants of the largely abandoned hopes of the Revolution, representing a national commitment to at least the promise (if not the reality) of health care as a universal right of the people.

As a response to the deficiencies of the system, a highly contested and deeply politicized package of reforms was introduced in 2001. Known as Seguro Popular or Popular Health Insurance, its stated aim has been to universalize public health access for the poor by shifting the federal budget to demand-based allocation, by separating purchaser and provider, and by integrating subsidies by federal and state governments along with premiums paid by families to insure against risk and medical impoverishment. It was initiated by Julio Frenk, health minister during the presidency of Vicente Fox and, problematically, designed, implemented, and evaluated by one and the same body of external, international health experts (Frenk et al. 2006).

The reforms were the subject of controversy. With little independent analysis of their effects, Frenk and his team, supported by the World Health Organization (WHO) and the *Lancet,* have claimed that Mexico is close to providing universal healthcare coverage, with Seguro Popular hailed as *the* example of health reform for low- and middle-income countries to follow (Knaul et al. 2012). These claims are contested and regarded by some as a corrupt and pernicious move by Mexico's neoliberal elite to mask their attempts to engineer greater market competition at the expense of the poor (Eibenschutz, Támez, and Camacho 2008; Laurell 2011; Támez 2008).

The tensions at the core of these reforms (access versus marketization) are particularly clear in the case of kidney disease. Dialysis and kidney transplantation are not included as part of the treatments covered by Seguro Popular and, given the disproportionate impact CKD has on the poor, this means Mexican families face increased economic and social impoverishment in the absence of adequate support outside of charging regimes.[4] Organizational inequities thus overlay a critical public health problem. Moreover, while Seguro Popular has increased access for treatments for some conditions, such as hypertension, HIV (e.g., antiretroviral therapy), childhood leukemia, cervical cancer, and care for prematurely born babies, one cannot assume similarities of experiences across chronic conditions (Knaul et al. 2012). As a result, Seguro Popular has a marked presence in those health services run by the Ministry of Health, and so represents another important aspect of the background to this study. I will discuss Seguro Popular along with concerns relating to social insurance in chapter 3.

Against the background sketched above, health professionals often referred to endemic fragmentation in the healthcare system as militating against an integrated, nationally organized system for deceased donation. Deceased donor kidney allocation is, instead, the function of each hospital's internal Transplant Committee, even though all patients are reported to CENATRA (Centro Nacional de Trasplantes, the National Transplant Center) (Cantu-Quintanilla et al. 2011). CENATRA is mandated by the government to oversee the wait-listing of patients in the National Registry: the supervision of licensed centers that perform organ procurements and the institutions authorized to perform transplants.

As broached in the introduction, we can now, perhaps, better see why Mexico provides an exemplary context for studying CKD and the replacement technologies of dialysis and transplantation. It is not just the matrix of institutional practice within which it is framed, it is also the scale of the populations affected: CKD is among the leading causes of death in Mexico (Garcia-Garcia and Chavez-Iñignez 2018).[5] Diabetes is said to be responsible for over half of all incident cases and is considered the primary cause of CKD (Alegre-Días et al. 2017).[6] The second major cause, as explained previously, is categorized as "unknown". However, as attention shifts toward this new variant of CKD, so too does the etiological narrative of this condition.

Within the public hospital, both staff and patients speculated about the country's increasingly deregulated economic environment post-NAFTA, particularly in relation to the food and agri-industries, poor toxic waste management, unchecked use of pesticides, and environmental pollution. This residual "unknown" (Parsons 1940) represents an important category of reference in terms of sickness and the state in Mexico but also the potential for articulating a political etiology of chronic disease. The category "unknown" indexes state and market failures as well as social and environmental crises. It is increasingly bound up with and exemplifies the processes of economic and social change tied to the neoconservative policies of Mexico's right wing government.

Assessing the actual epidemiological burden of CKD is considered a difficult task, particularly across so called low- and middle-income countries. This is predominantly due to the absence of kidney registries and comprehensive monitoring data (Ayodele and Alebiosu 2010). Mexico is no different, and so it is no simple task to present a straightforward epidemiological story. While the country contributes to a number of international registries such as the Latin American Dialysis and Transplant Registry (LADTR) and the United States Renal Data System (USRDS), it does not have an integrated national kidney registry. Data reported through these registries is also acknowledged to be weakened by voluntary and inconsistent reporting (Cusumano, Guillermo, and Gonzalez-Bedat 2016). Most of the epidemiological data is extrapolated from Mexican populations living in the United States or from localized Mexican surveys (Paniagua et al. 2007).

The state of Jalisco, where this ethnographic study was conducted, is a major contributor of epidemiological data. It is home to two of the country's more successful transplant programs, both based in the public hospital system: one in IMSS, the other in Hospital Civil. Nephrologists working within these programs established the Jalisco State Dialysis and Transplantation Registry in 1993, the only one of its kind in Mexico. The registry has relied on efforts to collect information, where possible, particularly from the social security institutions IMSS and ISSSTE as well as the institutions belonging to SSA—the Ministry of Health in the state of Jalisco. This has gone some way to keeping the condition under epidemiological surveillance and to generate data indexing CKD and its treatments nationally and internationally (Garcia-Garcia et al. 2005). Medical staff suggest that formal data sharing between institutions is not easy due to what is often explained as the closed and corporatist character of their healthcare institutions—their "silo mentality" in public management speak. Although the registry has yet to be mirrored in other Mexican states, it is now claimed to have data on approximately 90 percent of the dialysis and transplant population accessing services in Jalisco (Garcia-Garcia, Renoirte-Lopez, and Marquez-Magaña 2010). Data collection focuses on patients at the start of dialysis treatments. At this point, a patient's social security or insurance institution is registered along with age, gender, etiology of renal disease, and initial treatment modality. Unadjusted incidence and prevalence rates are reported and data on the number of nephrologists and dialysis and transplant facilities is annually updated (for further information on the methods used by the registry, see Garcia-Garcia et al. 2005). CKD manifests the politics of registries: ways of understanding population health and their fraught entanglements with local, regional, national, and international governmental arrangements.

In light of all this, the significance of actually achieving a diagnosis, of coming to count as a patient, cannot be taken lightly. Diagnosis unlocks the therapeutic interventions that follow—testing, monitoring, modalities of dialysis, drug regimens, surgery, and so on—establishing, at base, the practical ground of transplant medicine. While little is known about sufferers of CKD outside of formal healthcare systems, and screening is still in its infancy, doctors assume that many more patients than recorded, particularly from poor rural and indigenous communities, simply die at home. Of those who actually manage to reach diagnosis, approximately half are believed to die within six months of dialysis initiation or their first visit to a nephrologist (Gutierrez-Padilla et al. 2010).

Despite its limitations, the Jalisco registry has provided a way of thinking about and articulating the inequalities of outcome between CKD patients with and without insurance in this state. This has, in turn, helped to provide impetus for further interventions aimed at reducing inequity, such as screening and prevention, but has not lent itself to raising the profile of more structural, economic, or political concerns beyond the perennial problem of resourcing and the fragmented nature of healthcare delivery (Garcia-Garcia 2005, 2010). In Jalisco, those without insurance suffer higher mortality, significantly lower acceptance rates onto renal replacement therapies, lower rates of transplantation, and lower levels of access to a nephrologist (Garcia-Garcia, Renoirte-Lopez, and Marquez-Magaña 2010). Social Security covers 55.68 percent of the population in the state and a further 5.85 percent are covered by civil service and private schemes.[7] While 40.78 percent are identified as having Seguro Popular, 18.83 percent are left without any coverage or benefits at all.[8] These figures, however, are attributed to those who have chosen to enroll in Seguro Popular. As Seguro Popular provides no coverage for renal replacement therapies, not all patients will register.

The renal program offered at Hospital Civil, aimed principally at those without insurance, is unique in Mexico. It houses the country's largest dialysis and kidney transplant center for the uninsured section of the population. It has been home to a living-donor program since 1990 and a smaller cadaveric program since 1997. Due to problematic institutional politics, issues that I return to in chapter 6, these programs have largely travelled along quite separate roads since their inception, although efforts have been made in recent years to foster greater integration.

The hospital has a small hemodialysis unit with capacity for approximately sixty patients, which is used for the most part as a back-up service due to its high cost. It relies primarily on a large peritoneal dialysis program facilitating, during the time of study, 227 patients. As mentioned above, peritoneal dialysis is carried out in patients' homes and so is cheaper for the health services because it passes on costs to Mexican families that would otherwise be borne by cash-strapped hospital and medical centers. Jalisco was no different to the rest of Mexico in its reliance on this technologically mediated trade-off.

The hospital suffers a shortage of nephrology staff and is reliant on residents and nurses to support the transplant program.[9] With few exceptions, medical staff also hold positions at IMSS and some have established their own private practices. They work across these private and public domains, moving patients between them. They effectively work two jobs to make money and, in so doing, provide an informal conduit between different providers and patients. Medical staff, as I will show in later chapters, are located and operate at the intersections of intensely fractured and informal routes to healthcare. Hospital Civil maintains its reputation for helping the poor by virtue of the "hidden" work of many of its committed medical staff, who will spend additional time bending bureaucratic arrangements or writing letters of introduction for their patients to get drugs, tests, and treatments for free or at a reduced price. It would, however, be a mistake to treat Hospital Civil as simply a poor person's hospital. As a teaching hospital, it is also a site of medical innovation and development, as indexed by the transplant program. Outside of its uninsured cohort, it attracts a substantial number of IMSS and private patients who come to the hospital in search of what many regard as being better quality and more timely care.

Hospital Civil is therefore an important nexus in local flows of patients, technology, capital, and power, a site where organs acquire a socio-political life and are made into marketable and traceable things. It is also a site where processes of commodification and marketization could be (briefly) interrupted, bypassed, and redirected and where the emergence and escalation of diseases like CKD can be tracked: traced back to their complex biosocial and biopolitical causes and forward to the equally complex consequences for the institutions of family, medicine, and welfare. I now move out from Hospital Civil—the local setting—to follow the lives of those who move through it, biographical trajectories inflected and "torqued" by CKD. Following these lives through their encounters with a local healthcare infrastructure presents an important opportunity to understand how those involved in the transplant project, particularly patients and their families, secure care.

PATIENTS, THEIR FAMILIES, AND THE CO-PRODUCTION OF TRANSPLANT MEDICINE

The desire of Mexican families to obtain a kidney transplant for their loved ones opens up myriad stories, each unique for the diverse trajectories of care-seeking and the particularities of each person's case. However, throughout the course of fieldwork and across the wide range of personal accounts collected, clear commonalities emerged around the restricted nature of access to organ transplantation, the common constraints placed upon patients and their families, and the work they were thus required to do. In what follows, I present data from an ethnographic case, drawn on as an exemplar of these common constraints and chosen for its capacity to typify the structural character of the family's experience. This is the case of Elena and her family.

Elena and Her Family

Elena was an eighteen-year-old transplant recipient. Like many other patients whom I interviewed, she was young and had received no medical explanation as to why she had developed kidney disease in her mid-teens. Like so many others, her kidneys were too small to biopsy when diagnosed with CKD. She received her transplant in March 2011. Cesar and I interviewed her in July of that year at the hospital, and the following August with her family in their home. When we first met her, she was lying in the nephrology ward. She had been there for twelve days, awaiting test results. Cesar and I were introduced to her by Ana, her nephrologist, who was clearly annoyed with what appeared to be Elena's lack of commitment to her healthcare. Elena had not been attending her post-transplant consultations and was not following the dietary advice given to her by her doctors. Now she had complications and a urinary tract infection. From Ana's point of view, the staff at the hospital had worked hard to support her quest for a new kidney, and she was worried that Elena was not taking her responsibilities seriously. Ana thought that Elena's family had the financial means to support her medical care, which added to her frustration, particularly as so many of the patients she regularly saw and cared for could not have made it this far.

Our next opportunity to meet Elena was at her home in a small town surrounded by maize fields on the outskirts of Guadalajara. Lupita, her mother, met us off the bus. It had been an hour and a half's journey, much of it over bumpy dirt roads. She greeted us warmly and walked us to her small, white single-story house at the end of the *pueblo* (town) (see figure 2). She put her hand in through a cracked window pane in the front door and opened it, taking us into an L-shaped open-plan living room with a kitchen to the left. Elena's family were clearly *not* a family of means. Though relatively spacious, the house was sparsely furnished. The ceiling and walls were badly cracked. The kitchen had a large gas cooker, a refrigerator, open shelves for food and, in front of a small window with protective iron bars, an extendable family table, which had been half-cleared from the morning's breakfast. This was a much-used family kitchen, untidy and busy, one which had supported a family of eleven children over the years, plus grandchildren. Elena's mother worked in the home, and her father in a nearby fiberglass factory.

At one side of the living room were two bedrooms, both curtained off, one with bunk-beds and a TV and the other with a double bed. There was an additional

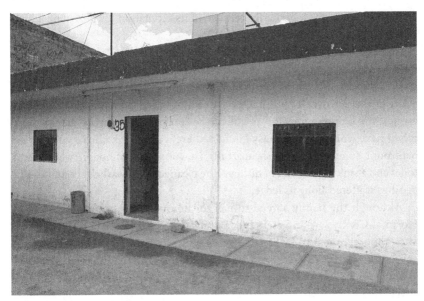

FIGURE 2. Elena's family home.

bedroom on the opposite side. This was Elena's room. It was also sparsely furnished. It had a large double bed, a small table with a TV and little else. The walls were white and the bedroom window was covered by a piece of pink floral material folded over to block out the light. In one corner of the room, spread across the wall, was a large stencil drawing of a tree with colored leaves. It was in this room that we were invited to sit and talk.

Elena's kidney had been donated by Rita, her older sister, who joined us for the interview. A mother of two small boys, she lived close by. Rita answered most of our questions, with occasional interruptions and clarifications from Elena and her mother. As chairs were brought in from the kitchen for us to sit on, Rita pulled out a large folder from behind Elena's bed, which contained all her hospital files, prescriptions, exam results, x-rays, and the like. With them all spread out on the bed in front of her, Rita proceeded to account for and illustrate the journey this family had taken to find and secure care for her younger sister.

Prior to diagnosis, Elena had experienced a range of symptoms: headaches, nausea, fatigue, among others. She had been to see three private physicians. Two diagnosed her with a throat infection; the third, on the insistence of her mother and sister, sent her for blood tests to a large public hospital in one of Guadalajara's municipalities.

Thinking that her symptoms might be linked to CKD, this doctor advised her to go to another public hospital, one supported by the Ministry of Health in Jalisco, because it provided free tests for poor people. But the family decided to go to

Hospital Civil instead, primarily because of its reputation for providing a high standard of care for families like theirs.

There, she was diagnosed with CKD. Her kidneys were at "end stage" and she needed dialysis immediately. She was prepared for peritoneal dialysis, so that she could have dialysis at home, but the catheter failed a number of times, and she was eventually put back on hospital-based hemodialysis. Looking around the family home, it was difficult to imagine how having dialysis here might have worked. In the busy kitchen, there was no sink. There was also no bathroom, so nowhere to wash, apart from a worn-out "out-house," which had a toilet and a sink already full of dishes to be cleaned, with washcloths and tooth-brushes scattered along its ledge.

Although the family agreed to pay for hemodialysis, the dialysis unit at Hospital Civil was completely full. Because Elena's parents had IMSS insurance, they were sent to IMSS facilities. As it turned out, Elena herself was not covered by this insurance. She had stopped attending school due to sickness and, now outside of formal state systems, she was excluded from the family's coverage.

For the next year and two months, she and her family would move continually between institutions in search of care. On the advice from one of the doctors at Hospital Civil, Elena and her family went to a small private clinic located in Libertad, a large working- class quarter of the city. The hospital provided dialysis at a relatively low cost of approximately 1,000 pesos (80 U.S. dollars), per session. One of the doctors in Hospital Civil, who had a working relationship with this private clinic, helped Elena to acquire a "discount" for the first few sessions, after which the family would have to pay the full costs of her three dialysis sessions per week.

While attending the small private clinic, the family, who were continually in search of financial support, were given a letter by one of the doctors working there to go to DIF Jalisco. DIF, Desarrollo Integral de La Familia, is a national charitable organization for families in need, and has federal, state, and municipal offices. In the DIF Jalisco state office, Elena received financial support for four free dialysis sessions. There they were given another letter to take to Caritas, Mexico, the international Catholic social welfare provider, where they got help paying for some more sessions. They then went to a DIF municipal office in Zapopan, who provided a little more support, and from there were sent to another DIF office in Guadalajara. Elena's mother, Lupita, took on the role of sourcing financial support. After three months of dialysis, they moved to SANEFRO, another private clinic run in conjunction with PiSA, a prominent Mexican pharmaceutical company that manufactures and distributes dialysis supplies. This they did with support from DIF Guadalajara.

When this support ran out, they were told of a local philanthropic organization and found support for eight further sessions. During this period—one year into

Elena's dialysis treatment—the family also made an "informal" arrangement with someone they knew who had a cleaning company to "hire" Elena so that she could qualify for IMSS insurance. The family, in turn, agreed to pay the employer and employee's insurance contribution.[10] With this in place, Elena received the remainder of her dialysis (two more months) free of charge at an IMSS-affiliated hospital. However, this was restricted to one session a week rather than the normally optimal three.[11]

Lupita had also applied for Seguro Popular on behalf of Elena, at the beginning of her illness, but was told it did not cover treatment for CKD or any of its medications. The family wanted to know if it could receive support for hospitalization expenses, but were told this was not possible. Seguro Popular did agree to cover consultations, which amounted to approximately 64 pesos (4.8 U.S. dollars) per session, but the family preferred to pay for this out-of-pocket to avoid the long queues that patients with Seguro Popular had to endure.[12]

Throughout her time on dialysis and despite the effort involved in securing access to it, the family, mostly through the efforts of her sister Rita, were simultaneously involved in looking for options for Elena to acquire a kidney transplant. They first tried with Hospital Civil, but because they had insurance, they were encouraged to go to IMSS. At IMSS, the family were told that while Elena was very sick, they could not do anything for her right away. IMSS, as the largest provider of care in Mexico, is known by patients to be notoriously slow, with long waiting lists. It would take more than a year just to get through all the protocols required for an organ transplant: the tissue typing, blood matching, and psychological tests needed prior to surgery. Distraught, the family went back to Hospital Civil to beg for a transplant. After extended negotiations, the hospital staff agreed to transplant her.

Before transplantation could proceed, the family had to pay for all the required pre-transplant protocols, many of which were outsourced to the new private laboratories that had sprung up around the perimeter of the hospital. Completing the protocols took almost eight months (approximately half the time at IMSS). In order to meet the costs, the family sold a small piece of land they had inherited, appealed to everyone they knew, requested money from relatives working in the United States, and went to local TV stations and businesses.

The price of histocompatibility (blood and tissue matching) tests in a private lab was approximately 1,400 pesos (112 U.S. dollars) each, for donor and recipient. In Elena and Rita's case, the tests had to be run twice, as Elena's initial tests were compromised because she had had dialysis-related anemia and subsequently had needed a blood transfusion. To help reduce the costs, on the second attempt, one of the hospital social workers sent them to a chemist she knew at IMSS who also worked independently in a private lab. Initially, they hoped that they would be covered by the new IMSS insurance they had set up for Elena but they were not. However, because the chemist worked on her own time, she charged them a slightly reduced amount of 2,000 pesos (160 U.S. dollars) for both donor and recipient tests.

Elena was eventually transplanted at a cost, for her surgery alone, of approximately 17,000 pesos (1,363 U.S. dollars). As a result of the expenses incurred, the family could no longer pay the contributions for IMSS, and as a result, Elena lost her insurance coverage. The family were forced to go to a money lender to get money for immunosuppressants. At this point, the family's resources had been so drained that they were finding it difficult to find the 475 pesos (38 U.S. dollars) for Elena to maintain her post-transplant monitoring and checkups, not to mention the 200 pesos (16 U.S. dollars) for the taxi fare to get there and back.

Unfortunately, Elena had complications post-transplant and an infection, and had to be rushed back into hospital. As the family explained, this was a result of overly tight surgical stitching that was restricting the flow of urine and had caused an infection. When we discussed Elena's case with one of the hospital doctors, we were told that the surgeon hadn't done a very good job.

One month later, we met Elena again in her family home. At this point, she hadn't returned for follow-up exams and consultations. The family were desperate. Rita, her sister and donor explained, "We are now *entre la espada y la pared* [between the sword and the wall]; we don't have money for Elena's post-transplantation care and don't have money to pay the money lender. We don't know what we are going to do."

IN SEARCH OF CARE: A PERPETUAL MOTION MACHINE

Stories other than Elena's could have been similarly used. All would have encompassed different waymarks, bringing their own pronounced difficulties; all would have exhibited the same tortuous structures; all would be underpinned by similar practices; and all would show the profoundly compromised but indispensable status poor bodies have within transplant medicine. In reviewing numerous case studies, the key point to note is how the lives and bodies of Mexico's uninsured kidney population are governed by movement.

In Elena's case, as in others, we see how movement underpins the process by which people make their way from falling ill to being diagnosed, to being treated on dialysis, to being put forward for transplantation and, from there, to what is euphemistically called post-transplant "care." This perpetual movement constitutes this population of kidney patients as families attempt to piece together a healthcare system for themselves: one created out of radical contingency and variability, out of fleeting encounters and the windows of opportunity for treatment they present across temporarily linkable sites, settings, and access regimes. This enforced movement tells of a logic of sickness and poverty that is both strict and unforgiving (Garfinkel 1984 [1967]; Lynch 1993). It is strict and unforgiving because it imposes discipline and hardship on those seeking essential healthcare for themselves and others. Moreover, in being so sequenced, the practices of the mobile poor link together and make visible the biopolitical character of organ transplantation in Mexico. Through the unpredictable lines of movement they must take to secure support, poor and sick bodies draw around them all manner of events, processes, and interactions that embody radically different kinds of exchange between very different kinds of actor. These include: gifts solicited and unsolicited; conditional and unconditional forms of support; social transfers in the forms of benefits and social insurance payouts; contractual obligations, barter, and monetary exchange; an unpredictably varied cast of agents; kinship and friendship networks, operating across national and transnational boundaries; state-level actors at federal, regional, and municipal level multiplied by the number of services provided: welfare, healthcare, education; supranational actors and expert knowledge employed for national and political interests; private sector actors—again fantastically varied: pharmacompanies, medical suppliers, laboratories, pharmacies, and the doctors who shift from being state actors to part of private enterprise depending on the manner in which they are approached; a multiplicity of civil society and non-governmental actors, but also employer networks, philanthropists, political parties, and the media; and the new science and technology capabilities which realize themselves in the presence of a growing transplant industry and the movement it necessitates.

The mobile poor operate without any overview of healthcare provision. Such infrastructures of healthcare lack the definable topology that would enable them to do so (Ruppert 2012). Unscripted, they make their way between various public and private healthcare providers, clinics, and laboratories. Without any social protection, families pay for everything—hospitalization, surgical procedures, routine check-ups and tests, dialysis, pre-transplant protocols, biopsy needles, stitching for wounds, disinfectant, antibodies, and medications. These payments must be borne on top of the costs of travel, food, housing alterations for home dialysis patients, informal caregiving, and the loss of formal earnings. Resources are obtained in different ways: by lobbying healthcare practitioners, medical practitioners, social care staff, corporations, the media; by the ad hoc payment of insurance premiums; by appeals to networks of family and friends; by selling land and inheritances; and begging.

In the absence of integrated administrative systems, patients and their families manage and carry all their hospital files, test results, and x-rays as they move between hospitals, pharmacies, and laboratories. As I saw on a number of occasions, patients would stand in the street or on crowded buses pointing to their files and appealing to their fellow citizens for financial help or food. Medical files are not held by any centralized bureaucracy. The patients themselves, not the state or any sited provider, are their own mobile archives, responsibilized social actors, the principal agent in the management of their healthcare.

Government by movement, such as this is, opens up some key questions and perhaps problems in drawing on a more standard or ideal-typical account of biopolitical regimes. Rather than being situated within an already definable apparatus of control—states, markets, medicine, welfare, systems of knowledge—which are brought to bear on visible constituencies and populations, the reverse is almost the case. Rather than functioning as the targets of these domains, as I go on to argue, the practices of the mobile poor are productive, indeed the organizational fulcrum, of these domains.

THE DISAGGREGATED POOR: PRODUCTIVE SITES IN THE MAKING OF MARKETS AND REGIMES OF POWER

In the absence of nationally organized kidney registries or an integrated epidemiology of kidney disease, its causes, treatments, or effects, we are reliant on ad hoc partial and opportunistic counting at local institutional levels. This leaves, at much broader levels, a disaggregated population, who are neither the objects nor subjects of discipline in a strict Foucauldian sense. Their status as "a population on the move" is an ambivalent one. As a population, they do not exist through enumeration; rather, a range of techniques, including enumeration, are parasitic upon their movement. Their movement provides the conditions of possibility for other types of opportunistic activity designed to capitalize on the cross-trade: new markets and new modes of governance.

CKD in Mexico marks out a somewhat different terrain of biopolitics than that which is conventionally advanced through technologies of calculation and administration, anchored in and constituted by the modern state (Estévez 2013; Foucault 2003 [1976], 1980). Still, in following Foucault's methodological precautions to trace the "real effects" of biopolitics at the "outer limits"—those points at which power becomes capillary and less juridical—we come to understand the varied ways in which subjectivities—modes in which individuals are treated as subjects of particular kinds—are produced as power-effects, as well as the particular power mechanisms that are brought into play for their production. For Foucault (2003 [1976]), by attending to the outer limits, where power is less unitary, where it transgresses the rules of right that organize it and delineate it, we stand to gain the most insight. In such sites, where lives are only partial objects of knowledge, never fully legible (Scott 1998), what happens does not simply have consequences for those who reside there, but also for the particular manner in which government via state and market, in turn, is constituted and its practices understood (Das and Poole 2004). These concerns are clearly exhibited by those who inhabit the margins of social welfare and entitlement in Mexico—such as Elena and her family—those with little choice but to act, to link up, and co-produce new markets and governmental configurations in medicine, as well as provide new ways of facilitating their operation.

The organs of the poor, frequently depicted in the anthropological literature as commodities, goods to be bought and sold (Scheper-Hughes 2000), can be seen in this context as work-sites for the extraction of surplus value, productive of new medical and pharmaceutical markets. As poor families move, as their bodies are worked on, they generate capital for others (scientifically, commercially, socially). Other commodities are dragged into orbit around them: dialysate solutions, catheters, antibodies, pharmaceuticals, laboratory testing, and the technologies of transplantation itself, put to work by variously involved parties (doctors, pharma companies, laboratories, and so on), all of which have to be paid for by families like Elena's. They pay to donate their "gift of life," which they then buy back through the services of transplant surgery, a process in which need is translated into market value, opportunities for others' labor and profit. The labor of Mexico's poor and sick renal patients not only generates surplus, but it does so in ways that make visible the governing strategies embedded in different forms of state and market practice.

Survival rates of transplanted organs are contingent on patients' capacity to pay for immunosuppression. The costs in every sense are high, not only in market terms but also in the gendered divisions that are produced as a result of the continual work families must do as they move in search of care. The transplant body rarely moves alone. Healthcare is a gendered problem with dual and specified configurations. In Mexico, gender differentiation is an explicit product of welfare regimes whose stratifying effects place women in evermore vulnerable positions (Esping-Andersen 1990). Gender inequity has been central to the aggressive processes of industrialization, post-NAFTA, which have transformed opportunities for financial independence into new sites of exploitation and violence, best seen through Mexico's expanding *maquiladoras* (factories) (Gaspar De Alba 2010). Mexico is thus characterized by what Haraway (1991) would call its own differentiated informatics of domination: disjunctures in the flows of goods, life chances, power, and government. These not only conscript women in new ways, but do so by laying claim to traditional forms of economic and gender cleavage, where women's roles—and bodies—are already culturalized as responsible for the "burden of caregiving" (DiGirolamo and Salgado de Snyder 2008) and made pivotal to the production and reproduction of family and social life.[13]

Following Spivak (2003), Elena's case helps us see the need to attend to occlusions of difference and what happens at the margins—of health, labor markets, welfare systems, and citizenship. These are sites where subaltern populations come to be produced and made productive, where those most central to the social distribution of responsibility are least resourced to see it through. And it is their action, crucially, which has an integrative role—a political role deprived, Spivak suggests, of all significance by analysts when their lives are read in purely structural terms. At the margins, therefore, regimes of power and government are increasingly exercised and the state remains a central force.

Regimes of power and government are neither abstract nor modulated but increasingly exercised through highly localized interfaces, as sites that must be negotiated for the next move to be made. These local interfaces will be drawn on to structure the following chapters in an attempt to map out a cultural anatomy of a biopolitical regime, an attempt to make visible those sites where the infrastructure of renal care is both produced and enacted. The discussions to come will pick up on recent thinking on the ways in which innovations in medical knowledge and technologies have been linked to shifts in state and market formations. For some, these processes are judged to be foundational to the rise of the biocitizen: the autonomous neoliberal subject, who exercises new frames of biomedical understanding to act upon him/herself (Rose and Novas 2005). This is not what is happening in countries like Mexico.

Changes in the production of surplus value have undoubtedly opened up the market-state-body nexus to new theoretical challenges and insights. Nonetheless, there are recognized and inevitable difficulties in drawing too heavily on what are, in effect, Anglo-American modes of understanding as guides for what might be happening elsewhere. When attending to the harnessing of the bios in the globalized south, Das (2001) argues that the potential for individuals to engage with or be engaged by varying forms of state and science cannot be assumed in advance, nor can we assume an inevitable logic in the management of life that operates uniformly across societies. If the conceptual framework of biopolitics is to be useful in understanding the relationship between life, power, and transplant medicine, the task is to find its relevance outside of Anglo-American welfare systems. We need to think about how its character alters across contexts. According to Race (2012), the intersections between state, market, and bodily health have yet to be worked through in ways that do not fall into problematically delocalized forms of critique, or take for granted the idea that neoliberal shifts in market activity automatically presuppose a rolling back of the state's role (Das and Poole 2004).

With that in mind, to say that contemporary forms of capital produce new forms of disenfranchisement is to say nothing particularly new. Rather than remaining at the level of general observation, we need to understand the sites and social practices through which human suffering is produced, in order to explicate how—in this case—renal care, capital, and the markets that operate in tandem with it have become so entwined when we interrogate their existing forms.

Labor, capital, the state, and politics are immediate presences in the lives of people touched by regimes of renal care. Insofar as the consolidation of such care *is* the elaboration of a biopolitics, these factors retain significance, albeit in a reconfigured manner. That Mexico's uninsured pinball between forms of healthcare provision in an attempt to establish bespoke arrangements of care provides us with an understanding of biopolitics that is situated and temporal. The manner in which uninsured patients sacrifice themselves and their limited resources to support a system that only benefits them in highly qualified and structurally ambivalent ways is itself a guide to the socio-political arrangements that both put them on the move and are constituted in their movement.

3 · LABOR
Producing Sickness and the State

        In Mexico, as in many other countries around the world, labor mar-
ket position is the key determinant of access to social insurance and sets the terms
and levels of entitlements to social protection and welfare. Entitlements typically
fail to deliver even minimum standards of support to those in need. In an increasingly flexibilized labor market, citizens move through various forms of work
with the same precarity they do various forms of healthcare. With health insurance as transient as labor market status, it is regularly lost through redundancy or
(re)gained in circumstances where patients have managed to come to informal
arrangements with local employers. At times, as discussed in the previous chapter, families abandon their health insurance in the face of bottlenecks, long waits,
or dissatisfaction with services, choosing instead to pay out-of-pocket to facilitate and quicken access to care due to pressing need. Under these conditions,
social security is to some degree always insecurely anchored, temporary, and
revisable.

    Existing scholarship on the state, welfare regimes, labor, and citizenship (Aretx-
aga 1997; Ferguson 1994; Gupta 2012; Ong 1999; Petryna 2002; Scott 1998) provides an important resource for understanding the situation of those who come
into contact with regimes of renal care, by showing how the emergence, consolidation, and organization of Mexico's hybrid corporatist/neoliberal welfare state
shapes their possibilities and life chances. Whatever claims are made on its behalf
"on paper," Mexico's welfare state is a perpetual work-in-progress. A governmental *autoconstrucción*; elements are continuously being adapted, added to but rarely
adequately finished as an outcome of political move and counter-move.[1] In practice, it works to lock large sections of the country's poor and economically insecure out of social security entitlements. This is partly due to a growing reliance
on new private markets in healthcare and their accompanying infrastructures,
which splice public and private provision.[2] However, while social and political
studies of the welfare state are valuable in sketching the contours of these kinds
of problems and their systemic bases, ethnographic research analytically deepens

and extends our understandings of them in crucial ways. In this chapter, I will show how it does so, by focusing on the ways in which patterns of inequality extend from particular forms of welfare, giving rise to a healthcare system increasingly dependent on the cash nexus and a limited social rights agenda.

THE CASE OF MARIA DEL ROSARIO

Maria del Rosario is in her early thirties, a single mother of two children; the oldest six years old. Her family live in Balcones de Sol among a group of *autoconstrucciónes*: family homes built over time by family groups, with extensions added as and when they are needed. Balcones de Sol is a poor barrio in the otherwise relatively well-to-do area of Zapopan, a city in its own right, though part of the wider metropolitan area of Guadalajara. Like many other poor barrios, it has expanded the margins of Guadalajara beyond the western Periférico, a sixty kilometer ring road that encases the city's outer limits, hemmed in by the rolling hills of El Colí. The land upon which Balcones de Sol now sits had in the past belonged to peasant and indigenous communities. Once used to raise corn and animals, the rights to it have long since been sold to developers and to the families who now live there. Through this process urban life has slowly encroached on land surrounding Guadalajara. Where families had once lived in relative self-sufficiency, they are, today, linked together in makeshift communities, characterized by intensifying precarity, sub-standard housing, and the growing salience of a *narcomenudeo*— the buying and selling of illegal drugs on a small scale as part of the local economy. The presence of this thriving local drugs trade could be seen throughout the neighborhood, with territories marked out by gang-related murals painted on the gable ends of houses (see figure 3).

Sitting in the small patio outside her parents' house (see figure 4), Maria explained that she had, in recent years, become the main caregiver for her mother Lourdes, a sixty-year-old woman with diabetes whose kidneys were in the final stages of functioning. The interior of the family home was only partially visible due to the sheets of tarpaulin it was shrouded in, helping to shield the family from newly begun renovations. These were largely the efforts of Maria's father, who was working to replace the mud floor with tiles and build an indoor bathroom, as part of the requirements for initiating CAPD (continuous ambulatory peritoneal dialysis) in the home. All that was visible when looking in through the open windows were various pieces of household furniture stacked against the walls; other pieces were temporally moved to the limited outdoor patio space in front of the house. Here we sat on a sofa with Maria, discussing her mother's health: "My mother was never sick or at least she never complained. It all started with her coughing. We gave her herbal teas and traditional herbs. We never imagined that her lungs were filling up with water. She didn't have many other symptoms. She did have cramps in her feet, but they were not swollen. She wasn't dizzy. She didn't

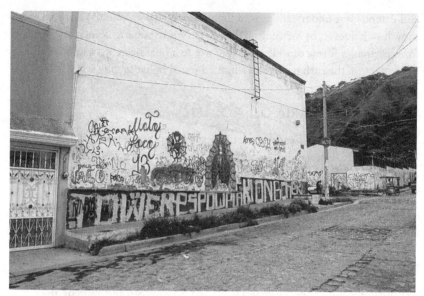

FIGURE 3. Local gang murals in Balcones de Sol.

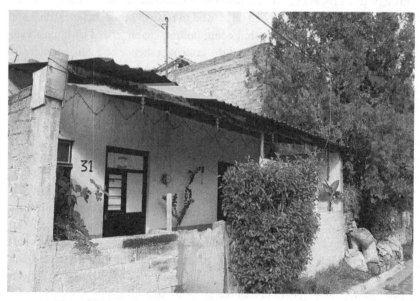

FIGURE 4. Maria del Rosario's mother's house.

have diarrhea, but in the last two days before she was diagnosed, water was coming out of her nose."

With her kidney functions nearing their end stage, Lourdes was told she would need dialysis imminently. Learning of this diagnosis was a source of intense frustration for Maria and her family. They had been trying to get to the bottom of their mother's symptoms for quite some time and—like Elena's family in chapter 2—this entailed endless visits to public and private clinics and hospitals.

In the two years leading up to diagnosis, Lourdes had various bouts of sickness. Although most of her symptoms were relatively unspecific, Maria felt that the medical attention her mother received had been far from adequate; securing it had largely been an outcome of the family's persistence. In the beginning, Maria explained, they brought their mother to the *hospitalito* (the name locals give to a small tertiary hospital in Zapopan) and from there, they were referred to Hospital General de Occidente in Zapopan (a hospital of the Ministry of Health, Jalisco). It had no space for Lourdes and the staff advised her to go to Hospital Civil to have medical consultations. She could not be admitted there, however, due to lack of bed space. The family had little option but to take Lourdes to a private hospital where she was put on medication to dissolve kidney stones and where, soon after, they learned she had diabetes. This was particularly aggravating for the family, because, as with many Mexican women of her age and class, Lourdes had been enrolled in Oportunidades, a social assistance initiative that includes a health promotion program with monthly medical check-ups, including monitoring for hypertension and diabetes.[3] No one had identified Lourdes's diabetes.

Lourdes was eventually diagnosed with CKD, following a three-day stay in the emergency room at Hospital Civil. Once diagnosed, she was hospitalized for three weeks in the *salas* before being admitted to the nephrology department to be treated with intermittent dialysis.[4] At this point, preparations had begun for dialyzing at home.

Despite the long road taken to obtain a diagnosis, there was no formal record of the journey the family took to get there. The haphazard route they took via a swathe of public and private providers would ensure little by way of accumulated paperwork to account for their efforts, their doctors' efforts, or even their mother's progressively deteriorating condition. But more important for Maria was what would happen next. They wondered what the future held in store for them, given the enormous challenges they were now to face trying to support a family member with CKD. She continued,

As a family, our entire world fell apart. It was distressing. We didn't know what to do or where to go for help. I almost went crazy. *None* of us have "formal" jobs—and, therefore, no way to pay for my mother's care. I also had to give up my part-time job as a cleaner to care for my mother. I feel traumatized that this can be happening to us; the work involved is overwhelming. I send my boy to school early in the morning, before 8 A.M., then go straight to my mum's house, come back when school is over, and then back again to my mum's house. I am continually moving backwards and forwards between houses. It is like working double-time, always. And I feel I have to keep my eyes open all the time for anything that might happen, particularly around medication and watching out for how my mum is feeling. I have to be prepared for everything. Up until now, my mother never took medication, not even a pill for a headache and now, suddenly, there are lots of pills and some of them seem to make her so sick. Twice, while in hospital and then soon after coming home, she threw up—but when she is back at home, she recovers. My mother is suspicious of the hospital and I really have to be vigilant. I don't feel I can ever trust what is happening.

Because the only treatment option for Lourdes was to have CAPD, a family member or caregiver had to agree to take the associated training to ensure that the treatment regime could be appropriately conducted at home. To aid a description of what this involves, I draw on Cesar Padilla-Altamira's ethnographic study of CAPD (2017) among the same CKD patient cohort in Jalisco. As Padilla-Altamira explains, CAPD patients are required to fulfill a training program, sit a related exam, and set up a dedicated *cuarto de diálisis* (dialysis room) in their homes. This room has to be prepared according to strict standards to minimize infections, particularly peritonitis. This includes constructing a floor out of polished cement or tiles (something that will not gather dust); ensuring that walls and ceiling are plastered and painted with a clear-color oil-based paint; that windows are sealed; that the door to the room is kept closed to prevent drafts and the accumulation of dust; and that the room is well lit. Inside, the room must include a bed (noting that the room can also double as the patient's bedroom); a table (50 cm × 100 cm recommended) with a clear surface, ideally a stainless steel surgical table; a washbasin; a twelve-liter jug and a water dispenser; a medical stand hook; a coat stand, or at least, a large nail on the wall on which to hang the dialysate bags; a microwave oven, to warm up the dialysate solution; and a scale to weigh the drainage bags at the end of the procedure. In addition, all families need: three scrub gowns; three scrub hats; one pack of disposable medical face masks; one plastic bowl of about 50 cm diameter; one thermometer; one re-usable soft brush (to wash their hands); one pack of regular or microfiber cloths; one pair of plastic clamps; one bottle of povidone-iodine; one bottle of hydrogen peroxide; one bottle of ExSept, a sodium hypochlorite, 50 percent disinfectant solution produced by the Mexican pharmaceutical company, PiSA. All in all, the construction of the *cuarto de diálisis* transforms the home into what Padilla-Altamira describes as a "para-clinical space," one that then has to be formally approved, with the patient providing photos to demonstrate that the required changes have taken place (Padilla-Altamira 2017).

The critical importance of the *cuarto de diálisis* for Lourdes's care was the reason that Maria del Rosario's father was renovating the family home. On the day of our interview with Maria, the house was still a long way off from conforming to the minimum standards and requirements set by the hospital. As her mother's main caregiver, Maria had already embarked on the CAPD training program. She could not, however, supply the photographic evidence of the house's suitability for home dialysis, to show it had adequate space, the necessary equipment, and met minimum standards of hygiene. Instead, to keep things moving forward, she "lied," submitting photos of a bedroom in one of her aunt's houses, in the hope that it would have a better chance to meet the hospital's requirements.

Over and above the physical and material preparations for CAPD, Maria found the training program and requisite exams intense and difficult.

> I thought I would pass the training, I was doing everything well. The nurses at the hospital told me I was ready, but I failed the exam that all new caregivers must take. I failed two questions because I was so nervous. After the exam, I was then expected to go for an interview but had no money to travel to the hospital. I wanted to call the nurses to explain my situation but didn't have a number for them. It was hopeless. I didn't have money and didn't know what to do. I didn't want to tell my mother too much about this, in case she worried, and her blood pressure rose. We are all having a difficult time financially. I've talked to my brothers, but they don't have any money, particularly to refurbish the house for dialysis. In my parents' house, there are no tiled floors, the doors are not in good condition and the walls are not plastered or painted. There is no money to change these things and this is why my father is trying to do it by himself.
>
> We also have very little money to pay for travel to the hospital and are constantly having to decide what *not* to buy, in order to pay for healthcare. We need money for dialysis treatments every two weeks. This is something which is necessary, but which my mother is reluctant to do, because she knows it costs so much and, of course, there are the additional tests and consultations that come with it.

If treatment is to be remotely sustainable, meeting the financial demands imposed upon families by a diagnosis of CKD means trying to negotiate lower costs with the hospital social workers. The social workers have an important mediating role when it comes to waiving or reducing costs associated with training, consultations, and hospitalization, sourcing cheaper medications, or in bringing forward hospital appointments. These negotiations are a fraught and contingent set of human interactions and success depends on the capacities of families to present a good case and provide documentation, as well as on the quality of relationships that the social workers themselves have with the various clinical specialties and individual medical staff. Given the recurrent and often unpredictable nature of medical costs, these fragile and contingent relationships are of critical importance.

Additional strategies to fund treatment also have to be employed depending on the means and capacities of individual families. For Maria and her family, aside from continually searching for the most cost-effective options, this included organizing *rifas* (raffles) to raise money in their local community. Maria's family were all traditional musicians and they relied on playing in public to supplement their income as laborers and cleaners. To support his wife's deteriorating condition, Maria's father had to first sell his accordion and then many of his laboring tools. The family then sold their TV and an electric piano. Selling the TV meant that they could cover some of the transportation to and from the hospital; selling the piano helped to cover their first two nephrology appointments and hospital stays. Her brothers regularly pawned their instruments when money was needed and they all pawned jewelry at various times. When money was needed urgently, they relied on a local money lender, but then had to cope with interest payments on these loans. All of this plunged the family into spiraling debt while simultaneously and systematically depriving them, through the loss of their instruments and tools, of the means to repay it, making them more, not less, dependent on external financial support.

Over the period Lourdes was ill, the family tried to access both social insurance (i.e., employment-based entitlements) and social assistance (i.e., poverty alleviation programs for those with incomes that fell below a means-tested minimum). Because Maria's father had two jobs, he had two social insurance numbers and cared for his wife through IMSS on that basis. But help was difficult to secure that way, due in part to the instability of laboring work but also due to the long waiting lists for treatment associated with IMSS. Lourdes did have access to Seguro Popular, but, as I explained in chapter 2, apart from providing some financial support to cover the costs of tests and medications, it did not support treatment for CKD.

For Maria, the burden of care and worry, of waiting and negotiating, of having to maintain constant vigilance for the health of her mother, fell squarely on her shoulders:

> It is so difficult. I am a single mum and it was hard for me to stop working. I thought, how am I going to support my children now? My siblings told me that they were going to help me, and they have done some things, like buy stationery for the children for school, but we are struggling—right now I can't afford books for my daughter. Life has always been difficult, but I coped before. Now I don't know what to do, because so many things are happening suddenly and without warning—and there is just no choice but to deal with it. I feel traumatized—what is happening is overwhelming.

FORMS OF LABOR, FORMS OF WELFARE

The struggles of families like Maria's are lived out at the unstable interface of forms of work—in particular, insecure work—and forms of welfare and social protection. At these interfaces, the role and responsibilities of the state to its citizens come explicitly into view and the biopolitical arrangements of renal care are acutely articulated. To tease out the associations between the state and transplant medicine, I focus attention on Mexico's welfare arrangements as they are encountered by people who are poor and uninsured, like Maria and her family, as they seek treatment for CKD.

In doing so, I address the idea of labor in two mutually informing ways: (1) in relational terms, examining the vulnerable and insecure position poor and casualized workers have within the Mexican labor market and (2) in terms of Arendt's notion of labor*ing* or toil and its connection to bios or life when it comes to CKD in contemporary Mexico. This is the unending labor that is required from the poorest and most insecure if they are to live when forms of waged labor do not insure against the risks of sickness and when the state's apparatus of social protection not only fails but renders their situation markedly more difficult. This failure of social protection gives rise to profound "dispossession," both in the classical, historical, and political-economic sense, such as where a landed peasantry, stripped of their rights to the land, is made dependent on waged labor and the cash nexus, generating a property-less proletariat with little control over or access to the means of production (Marx (1974 [1867])) but also in the sense that state failures to ensure adequate compensation, within a market economy under the wage-labor relationship, for loss of earnings via welfare entitlements and protections, dispossess the poor of the means to sustain and reproduce life at its most fundamental. In such circumstances, where the non-market forms of social reproduction necessary for participation in the market are themselves commoditized, life becomes a metered good, payment for which threatens continued living. This can be seen in particularly stark terms when it comes to CKD. Inadequate compensation mechanisms have profound consequences in the context of a condition, where dependence on technological medicine *is* the only means to live, and where attempts to access it not only threaten the survival of individuals but also those they are bound to: their families.

Such intensified downward spirals of neglect and harm might also be said to be antithetical to the long-term project of "capital" itself (Esping-Andersen 1990). As capital spreads out ever more deeply to invest the very social relations that provide its preconditions, it destabilizes them and makes them untenable. In a de facto state, described by Engels as "social warfare" (1926 [1845], 25), the capacity for capital to reproduce itself may also therefore be severely damaged, particularly when the state has progressively abandoned the socially and economically reparative roles it may once have claimed. The cannibalization of the social by the economic is, thus, far from implication free, generating markets grounded in highly specific forms of human sacrifice. In emphasizing the ambivalent project of welfare, and by showing the ways it has become bound up with the production of penury, attempts to harness the work of labor result in ever-more injurious outcomes and a state-regulated sacrificial economy around healthcare. In this, I contend, we are witnessing a "remaking of the social" (Latour 2005) via a biopolitics of indifference.

One of the key questions driving my analysis in this chapter is how to understand a healthcare system that produces hardship and harm rather than health. It is tempting to read the challenges faced by families like Maria's in purely structural terms (i.e., to see these social and health inequalities as an outcome of capital or recent waves of what are now typically, but perhaps misleadingly, labelled neoliberal policies, policies that have served to amplify rather than ameliorate the plight of the already precarious poor).[5] No one would wish to deny, for example, the stratifying effects of healthcare systems when those who turn to them are dependent on the cash nexus for access to services. We could, as a result, read the harms inflicted upon the lives of the most vulnerable as a form of structural violence and tease out the specific ways in which the social institutions of health and welfare, the Mexican state itself, produce an unequal distribution of harm. However, as ethnographers, we remain sensitive to the analytical limits of such master categories (state, capital, and so on) as things that bear down on people, enabling or constraining their possibilities in pre-determined ways. As these master categories are extended to cover a wider and wider range of contexts, processes, and outcomes, they become incapable of distinguishing between them, flattening out important differences. How harms are locally mediated, how they diversify and spread, can drop from view if we move too quickly to the level of general structures. In making invisible the specificities of power and its effects, such explanatory devices can reify the determinants of poverty and its harms. They tell us that power is structural and that the state and its actions are "relatively" autonomous and so analytically separable from the stratified lives of its citizens, on whom it acts without caching out the terms in which this occurs in any particular case (Burawoy 2000; Tsing 2009).

A particular problem with "top down" structural accounts is that we come to see what happens to those who are poor merely as a produced effect. However, as an alternative, we might consider, following Foucault, what it would mean to treat the situations of families like Maria's as productive in and of themselves. What I mean to draw out, by casting things in this way, is that the changing conditions of a political economy put the lives and livelihoods of those most vulnerable in jeopardy. This serves to re-make and refashion capital-social relations by putting the onus and responsibility for managing them on those most directly affected. What we see in the case of Maria's family are circumstances where individuals have to break themselves and one another continually as part of situationally creative responses to the radical contingencies of their situations. Through the informal practices of debt management, through the enforcement of new solidarities, or through the sacrifices required of extended family and networks of friends, Mexico's uninsured put themselves to work. In the course of that work, they forge the material bases for new structures and relationships to emerge.

To anchor this argument, I build analytically from the ground up. A starting point for doing so is the problematic status of the sick and chronically ill especially, within capitalist societies, something that forced itself on the attention of Talcott Parsons, among others, and to which he returned several times. Parsons was struck by the disruptive character of sickness, its capacity to threaten normative orders and the functional integration of individuals in society. All societies would have to develop ways of dealing with the problem of sickness, of absorbing it and taming it, but it took a particularly acute form in societies with a moral economy defined by wage-labor relationships. Where normative expectations say that an individual must work to live and access social support, being unable to work places an individual outside the moral order. The solution devised was to provide a controlled space that would enable a return to normality, preferably through recovery and rejoining the workforce or by subjection to arrangements within which an inability to recover would be continuously certified and recertified—Parsons's venture into the Foucauldian territory of the disciplinary and the governmental. Sickness was thus "allowed"—there could be life without work—but it was also constrained, institutionalized, and rendered manageable through these arrangements and the "sick role" they established.

What we see in contemporary Mexico's approach to the management of chronic illness and its treatment is a very different moral economy of care than the mid-century U.S. system examined by Parsons in developing his analysis of the sick role. In the United States, control of the sick not only included conferring rights on them but also particular obligations. In this way, they would not have to participate as productive members of society but would instead be supported, provided they observed certain rules, through the joint maintenance of a status he referred to as "sanctioned deviance" (Parsons 1951). Parsons's sick role was thus rooted in an institutionally supervised system of reciprocity and recognition with allocative and distributive consequences that emerged as a function of a particular kind of capitalist society and its defining forms of economic and non-economic exchange at a particular moment in its history (Varul 2010). A stabilizing institutional bridge of that kind between the sick and society, through a specific configuration of welfare, was essential if that particular form of capitalist society—the full employment, growth-oriented, expansionist economy that emerged post-war with its corporate paternalist moral order—was to be maintained (Blane 1987; Varul 2010).

That type of society has, of course, subsequently been politically and economically deconstructed. Nonetheless, Parsons's analysis of it contains much we can still learn from. While the deterioration of that particular institutional bridge might be thought to cast doubt on the value of Parsons's analysis, we should be wary of thinking his account of the "sick role" was ever intended to be invariable or indefinitely extendable. As a solution, a functional response, the arrangements Parsons analyzed were historically situated. As the arrangements that define social, political, and economic relations shift and change—particularly welfare arrangements spanning both the public and private sectors and family, community, and civil relationships—so will the moral relations that underpin, structure, and make consequential recognition of the position of the sick. As Varul (2010) points out, different ways of organizing and responding to the structure of the social relations of capital and waged labor fundamentally change what it can mean to be sick both within societies over time as well as across different societies at the same time. In the Mexican case, sickness itself is turned into an "occupation," a form of labor in its own right. There is no escape from work even when participation in the labor market in return for wages is no longer a possibility. However, to extend Varul's argument further, it is worth pursuing what else this antagonistic way of ordering relations and the social recognition of the sick might be doing, what else gets produced in its wake?

To answer these questions, in their specific forms in specific places, neither capital nor the work of the welfare state (nor the social expectations and obligations that are conferred on the healthy and the sick) can be taken for granted or assumed, something the comparative project of anthropology bears out (Aretxaga 1997; Ferguson 1994; Gupta 1995, 2012; Scott 1998; Navaro-Yashin 2002). One thinker who makes full use of this comparative lens, though not an anthropologist, is the Danish sociologist Gosta Esping-Andersen (1990), in his work on the political economy of welfare. In examining the internal logics and historical genealogies of welfare regimes, varying "worlds of welfare capitalism," Esping-Andersen emphasizes how very different ways of practicing capitalism produce very different modes of social stratification. Working with an "ideal" typology of democratic, conservative, and liberal worlds of welfare capitalism, Esping-Andersen shows them to be not merely descriptive of different forms of welfare but key to understanding the causes and socioeconomic consequences of these differences (Korpi 2000). Welfare systems, he contends, cannot be treated as mere functions of capital and the state, but are themselves outcomes of particular labor market histories, ongoing political conflict, and struggle and the shifting balance of power within a society between labor, capital, and the state over time. At root, welfare states embody histories of political struggle, played out on a terrain established by the political struggles of the past.

While offered as a reflection on European polities, Esping-Andersen's typologies have been drawn on to investigate different social policy approaches in Latin America. Despite recognition of the value of Esping-Andersen's emphasis on processes of stratification and commodification in analyses of welfare outcomes, there has been little consensus among scholars as to how one should best characterize the additional social policy clusters that have emerged across Latin America over the course of the twentieth century (Barrientos and Hinojosa-Valencia 2009; Filgueira and Filgueira 2002; Martínez Franzoni 2008; Schneider and Soskice 2009). In the context of Mexico, Esping-Andersen's work attunes us to welfare as a very particular product of social, economic, and political history—of post-revolutionary restructuring and state modernization. The contours of this history are well-rehearsed across social policy and sociological literatures (Brachet-Márquez 2007; Murai 2004; Mesa-Lago 1978) and provide an important starting point to understanding the situations and challenges that Maria and people like her confront.

THE GENERATION OF SYSTEMIC FRAGMENTATION

I want to briefly emphasize those features of Mexican welfare and its development that help us to account for the dysfunctions and harms we see manifest in the case of CKD. The rise and development of the welfare state in Mexico,[6] as in Latin America more broadly, is not one that can be said to reflect a single logic.[7] Its particular form was driven by very different arrangements and historical circumstances to those in Western and Eastern Europe, where industrialization, the subsequent demand for labor rights, and the process of democratization led to demand for, and the growth of, protections from the risks of market participation via the development of the welfare state and generalized systems of social entitlement (Brachet-Márquez 2007).

Up until 1982, the Mexican welfare state was characterized as a limited conservative corporatist regime, involving institutionalized brokerage and thus cooperation between capital, labor, and the state on behalf of social stability. This system of brokerage and cooperation has its roots in the Cardenas government of the 1930s.[8] Cardenas wanted to make the country's largest labor unions the base of his party's support, and so promoted collective bargaining agreements that included social security benefits as well as wages (Mesa-Lago 1978). As a political strategy, this would become an engine of internal stratification based on the systemic favoring of vested interests, with other people—those already marginalized—locked outside systems of state support and ignored in attempts to extend them. For example, IMSS was established in 1944 as a contribution-based system financed through payroll taxes paid into by employees and employers, and was meant to provide coverage for the formal labor sector. However, the larger and more powerful unions, such as those in the petroleum and railway industries, expressed their opposition to joining, due to IMSS's comparatively low benefits, and opted to retain their own separate systems of entitlement (Murai 2004). The Confederación de Trabajadores de México (Confederation of Mexican Workers [CTM]), made up in the main of union organizations in small- and medium-sized companies, became the base of governmental support and the larg-est constituency of IMSS subscribers. Fragmented and incomplete, these new social security institutions had a lasting effect. Among other things, they privi-leged urban Mexico and strengthened the labor core, while marginalizing rural and indigenous populations who could not access these new systems. Those out-side of formal systems of entitlement would, instead, be reliant on the Secretaría de Salubridad y Asistencia (SSA) with its own Ministry for Health and network of subsidized, but underfunded, public health hospitals managed by the indi-vidual Mexican states. Rather than addressing social inequality, Mexico's sys-tems of welfare entrenched and amplified differences. People who were already advantaged were well served; those who were already disadvantaged struggled to access assistance. Various attempts over the following decades to make up for the limitations of an increasingly fragmented, dysfunctional, and unequal welfare state would be made, but with little success.

Segmented entitlement was, as a consequence, institutionalized by the Mexi-can welfare state and had its own idiosyncratic processes of social stratification—civil servants (and their dependents), differentiated from workers (and their dependents) in nationalized industries, from workers (and their dependents) in sectors where the big unions held sway, from workers (and their dependents) in sectors where unions were less concentrated, from the urban poor, from the rural poor, and from indigenous communities. This segmentation persisted and in, many respects, intensified after the global debt crisis in 1982, which saw this corpo-ratist model reshaped into hybrid liberal form, whereby the state's responsibility to its citizenry was largely abandoned in favor of minimum interference with market outcomes (Murai 2004).[9] At that time, as is the case today, more than half of the population had no social insurance coverage. Among the poorest, who still had not attracted the state's attention, were indigenous groups, whose existence was politically acknowledged after the Zapatista rebellion, too late to be included in a fast-dwindling welfare state.[10]

The deregulation of the market served the interests of Mexico's dominant class while wages declined for average Mexican workers. By 1997, middle-class work-ers earned only four times the amount considered to be a poverty-level wage (Portes and Hoffman 2003). The number of households below the official pov-erty line increased from 34 percent in 1970 to 43 percent in 1996 (Shefner 2008). As was the case elsewhere in Latin America, social inequalities in Mexico wors-ened considerably from the 1970s onward (Boltvinik 2003), bringing an increase in migration to urban centers. This shift led to the proliferation of communities, like Balcones de Sol where Maria and her family live, at the periphery of Mexi-co's towns and cities. These communities are characterized by substandard hous-ing and limited public services and social support. Anti-poverty measures to curb social inequality have expanded in tandem with the very structures of welfare that are paradoxically implicated in the rise of such inequality in the first place.

Oportunidades—the program that Lourdes, Maria's mother, was enrolled in (and that failed to identify her failing health)—is one of the better known.[11] Its purpose was to break the intergenerational cycle of poverty—previously identified by Lewis (1961)—by operating a conditional cash transfer (CCT) program.[12]

As Enrique Valencia Lomelí (2008, 477) points out, "depending on whom one credits, CCT programs, like Oportunidades, represent either a daring new approach to fighting poverty, one that respects market principles . . . or a stripped-down approach in a region dominated by a minimalist social policy . . . For some observers, CCT programs stand for greater efficiency, whereas for others they constitute a reduction in the commitment to social justice, one that focuses only on the most extreme cases of poverty." The presence of such programs is not, however, a peculiarly Mexican phenomenon; it represents a continuation of broader economic reforms in Latin America that have sought to develop instruments of social policy that reflect wider market logics. The "conditional" aspect of their operation is an individualized one, driven by an ethos of behavior change based on an assumption that, rather than being recipients of redistributive state action, individuals should break cycles of intergenerational poverty. Neglected in all of this is any consideration of the structural forces at play and the practices that ground them (i.e., the importance of labor market demands and the provision of economic opportunities in contexts of hardship).

The effects of Oportunidades are difficult to ascertain, and attempts to do so have depended on evaluating enrollment and attendance numbers rather than the quality or practice of provision itself. For Valencia Lomelí among others, a persistent challenge for this initiative, as with initiatives that preceded it, is the extent to which such interventions can be integrated within existing social security institutions as a means to curb segmentation and the stratification of outcomes that goes hand-in-hand with it. Valencia Lomelí (2008) suggests that without an explicit commitment to strengthening social citizenship through guaranteeing rights and engendering stronger political participation among those most marginalized, little will be done to alter the fragmentation at the heart of the Mexican welfare state (see also Barba Solano et al. 2005; Barba Solano 2007).

Poverty is a vexed subject in Mexico, and it is not easy to establish a clear picture of its distribution across the population. Since the international banking crisis in 2008, there have been heightened concerns over further deterioration in the labor market and rises in poverty (Cantú Calderón, Gómez López, and Villarreal Páez 2016). The picture according to the available poverty statistics has been contradictory in several respects. In 2013, CONEVAL (Mexico's National Council for the Evaluation of Social Development Policy) suggested that Mexico's poverty rate had fallen slightly between 2010 and 2012, dropping 0.6 percent, from 46.1 percent to 45.5 percent, while the number of people living in poverty increased from 52.8 million to 53.3 million, due to population growth. Thus while poverty declines, the number of the poor increases (Wilson and Silva 2013). INEGI, the

Mexican-state-run statistics service (which reports to CONEVAL), has also claimed in recent years that Mexico's poor were richer by 33.6 percent, arguing an overestimation of previous poverty levels. The claims have been met with critical backlash from anti-poverty groups, who have argued that such figures were less a result of an improvement in the position of the poor and more due to changes in INEGI's methodology for measuring household earnings. This has attracted media attention inside and outside Mexico. David Agren (2016), writing in the UK *Guardian*, noted that the figures showed an overall increase of 11.9 percent in household earnings, with the poorest making the biggest gains, but added, "measuring poverty has proved controversial in Mexico, where social programs are often criticized as vote-buying exercises and beneficiaries in some states are told erroneously that their benefits are conditional on supporting the party in power." Reductions in poverty as officially measured may, therefore, be artifacts of politics in rather direct ways. This criticism has also been levelled at Seguro Popular and its stated attempts toward universalizing health and welfare provision for the poor (Laurell 2015).

BEYOND THE FORMAL ACCOUNT:
FOLLOWING THE PATIENT, FOLLOWING LABOR

The fragmented or segmented character of Mexican welfare invites the kinds of readings that imagine welfare arrangements to extend outward from particular types of political economy, mapped onto, in turn, different constituencies of the population. In other words, one can easily produce a formal reading of welfare and entitlement that takes its functions, coverage, and effects at face value, without recognizing that such readings are themselves endpoints in historical and political practice. As I have described in chapter 2, there are many gray areas within the system: loopholes, blind spots, anomalies, and openings that can be taken advantage of in the interest of securing faster, better, or cheaper care and support. The formal distinctions that appear to characterize welfare entitlement are artifices, useful institutionalized fictions. Superficial readings tell us very little about their uses and affects because their deployment is often an exercise in misdirection—the story is elsewhere. And in finding the story elsewhere, we also see that regimes of renal care, by extension, cannot be articulated via the rhetoric of segmentation. Instead, they are pulled into focus and extended by the various moves that Mexican families make. The zig-zagging routes and journeys taken by Elena's and Maria's families to secure care—in the absence of formal entitlement—demonstrate this. But so too, do the efforts of families who have access to insurance and who show up at Ministry of Health hospitals when the cumbersome and saturated services at IMSS prove too much to cope with. Laura and her husband Javier, an insured couple I met in Hospital Civil, exemplify the failures and breakdowns that arise even when social entitlements have been secured. I now turn briefly to their case.

Laura and Javier

When I met Laura, she was recuperating in an isolation room on the recently refurbished fourth floor of La Torre. She had received a kidney from a deceased donor the previous day. The calm of Laura's recovery room was in sharp contrast to the chaos of the nephrology ward one floor above. Laura and Javier also contrasted with the patients I normally met there. As IMSS beneficiaries, they were entitled to transplant care, though endured problems acquiring it.

Javier had a good job working for a construction company, which afforded IMSS insurance. However, he and Laura had been frustrated by their inability to access hemodialysis in IMSS hospitals due to the high demand for the service. In order to secure care, they paid out-of-pocket to Sanefro, a private clinic, spending all their savings in the process. Not only was Javier having to forgo his social security entitlements, he also had to increase his working day to between fourteen and sixteen hours to make the extra money they needed to pay for Laura's dialysis treatment. Soon after starting dialysis, Laura was put on the deceased-donor transplant waiting list, as she did not have a suitable living-related donor. This was five years prior to transplant surgery.

For Laura, these five years were positive. Her fellow dialysis patients were like a family to her—they shared experiences and traded *albures* (dark humor) about their fistulas, the dialysis equipment, and their failing health. Laura, who was forty years old (and Javier forty-seven) when we met, was diagnosed with diabetes twenty-two years before and knew that there was a risk she would develop kidney failure. As a consequence, the couple had no children and described themselves as a tight, protective unit.

Because of her diabetes, Laura and Javier were hoping that a double transplant (i.e., pancreas and kidney) would solve their problems, but the pancreas retrieved from the deceased donor was not of sufficient quality. At first, they were reluctant to only accept a kidney, but as they had waited so long, they felt they had little choice, fearing further deterioration in Laura's health. In looking ahead to life after transplant surgery, they were met with a new set of concerns (i.e., how to bear the costs of immunosuppressant medication). They asked their family and friends to help, as they had exhausted their savings. Javier said that he would go back to IMSS and demand the drugs they needed for immunosuppression. He said he felt betrayed having worked hard for so long paying money into his IMSS insurance for nothing.

What Laura and Javier, and Maria's family before them, show are the limitations, the futility of relying on any formal account of Mexico's welfare arrangements as an indication of who has access to what. Just because welfare arrangements are in place does not mean they work in the way they are said to or have been designed to. Despite differing points of origin, both Maria's and Laura's cases make clear that in order to unpick the practical functions of social entitlement, we have to turn to the people themselves: to their practices and what they are required to do. It is only in following their labor that we learn about the functions and dysfunctions of a welfare system. In doing so, we are drawn to the neglectful dispassion of Mexican welfare, as Mexican families are often faced with abandoning paid work (their only means of living)—or in Javier's case, extending it beyond his limits—in order to access renal care. In effect, Mexican families rely on a system that systematically destroys them and their means of surviving. It dispossesses them of the capacity to sustain life as they live and work against their own interests. The version of welfare we are left with here, in the case of CKD, is nominal. Rather than navigating a neatly apportioned system of entitlement and assistance, Mexican families wrestle with the wreckage of a system that has never found a stable ground. Within this wreckage, labor finds its meaning as families take up the work of the state.

The physical and emotional labor that this requires produces a downward spiral, one harnessed to the bodies, lives, and futures of citizens to perform welfare for themselves. The state bears little witness in return. As discussed in chapter 2, the provision of renal care produces a particular form of biopolitics, one that does not rely on the legibilities often enshrined in record keeping, hospital registries, and administration, where patient cases acquire a formal "social life" (Appadurai 1986). As a result, the "knowing" side of the welfare state is drastically underdeveloped and, to some extent, does not need to be otherwise. These "states of ignorance" (Rappert 2012), such as they are, allow the state to exploit the gaps in its own field of vision. What this shows is that state work, contra Scott (1998), is not always served by making populations visible and legible but can be served by the reverse, keeping them invisible and illegible. What is not known, with any certainty, need not be acted on. In supporting a state-society-market nexus that establishes the conditions of access to healthcare and provides the practical ground of renal care in this context, the invisible and illegible labor of Mexican families is central, just as it is to the production of a biopolitics through the elaborative work it performs. This is a situation in which the state puts the isolated individual and the extended family to work—that is, in facilitating the exploitation of one (the patient), it facilitates the exploitation of all (the family). In serving to disembed healthcare, particularly for those most reliant on it, the welfare state becomes not only an agent of penury, it operates in ways that are antithetical to life itself.

The ambivalence of welfare in Mexico, as its own genealogy shows, owes much to the cross-interference patterns that have come to define its growth and development over of the preceding century. The role of co-option and the bargaining power of elites and interest groups simultaneously characterize both the growth and dysfunctions of welfare. It has left some wondering whether the Mexican social contract is broken, given that the basic necessities of everyday living—health, housing, education, personal and public security—can no longer be said to be public goods, shared and maintained by all, but are linked to a regressively distributive politics organized around the inequalities of the cash nexus under wage-labor relations.[13] This has produced harm, neglect, and pathologies of care. Without fulfilling the functions of protection, the very attempt to secure welfare is killing Mexican citizens, dispossessing them of their labor power in the most fundamental ways, while yoking their efforts to pursue care to the workings of the state and market, and at the same time drawing many others into the oubliette in the process. Labor is, therefore, key to the remaking of social worlds. This remaking, I have suggested, is predicated on a biopolitics of indifference.

Outside of the implications this has for Mexico and its citizens, encountering a situation of this kind forces us to reflect on what might be changing within welfare states elsewhere: to ask to what extent the processes we see in Mexico are part of much broader global changes; and to what extent they are situated and specified. With the erosion of both the funding mechanisms of welfare states today, and their capacities to distribute and redistribute different types of social assistance and entitlement, there is little doubt that the architectures of modern welfare states are in trouble. We see this most acutely in those countries that once stood as a blueprint for other social systems, such as the UK and Sweden (Dalgren 2014; Pollack 2005).

Reflecting on the UK, in a recent review essay on Chris Renwick's *Bread for All: The Origins of the Welfare State,* Susan Pedersen (2018) makes clear that the creation of a universal welfare state is never simply a matter of enacting specific programs to meet specific social needs (despite this emphasis by successive Mexican administrations); it requires a prior commitment to economic management and a tolerance for state control of significant aspects of public life. Democratic welfare states, in other words, rest on democratic structures and values. They require that society be seen as "[a] whole, its members interdependent and solidaristic, subject to predictable processes or laws, and hence alterable . . . through social programmes and interventions" (5). The welfare state—its successes and its failures—is contingent on the particularities of political economy. Pedersen continues:

All advanced industrial societies became welfare states in the 20th century, even the anti-collectivist United States. All states came to collectivise risk to some extent; all tackled public health and poverty; all expanded the scope of public finance. But the particular risks states chose to address, and the programmes they developed to attack them, varied; and those programmes weren't necessarily "progressive". France was slow to develop comprehensive unemployment insurance but was a pioneer in addressing the costs of children's dependence; Nazi Germany showered benefits on families, but only when they promoted the regime's racial imperatives. Welfare policies meet social needs but they also construct social norms and inflict social punishments: they can foster as well as ameliorate distinctions or inequalities. Welfare states provide entitlements: but to whom, and in what form, and under what conditions? When it comes to welfare states, the devil is always in the detail.

The value of the ethnographic enterprise is in focusing attention on this detail. It is essential to understanding the infrastructures that ground regimes of renal care and that provide or deny access to them. Labor market position, in its interfacing with welfare and thus healthcare, provides us with one vantage point from which to pursue those details, showing us in the process, a remaking and refashioning of capital-social relations. The next chapter extends a consideration of the detail to the clinical encounter, examining a further set of interfaces through which access to renal care must be negotiated and through which it is materialized.

4 · BROKERING HEALTHCARE

Paper-work, Negotiation, and the Strategies of Navigation

Characterizing sickness and harm as extensions of state practice—or structural violence—raises important and difficult theoretical and methodological questions about what we are doing when we describe the state in this way. The work of a generation of ethnographers cautions against over simplification when discussing the state or attributing blame to a readily identifiable "it," a Leviathan, a thing in and of itself. Conceptual and methodological defenses are needed to avoid the temptation to misread abstractions as concrete truths. One useful strategy is to examine the state through its effects and how they are made manifest in specific sites and settings—those places where it can be practically shown to acquire significance in and for the workings of social and cultural life (Das and Poole 2004; Ferguson 1994; Ferguson and Gupta 2002; Gupta 1995, 2012; Sharma and Gupta 2006; Navaro-Yashin 2002).[1] In this chapter, I follow precisely this methodological path, focusing attention on the clinical encounter—the ordinary interface between patient and doctor (or other health professional). I examine the ways in which care for CKD and access to renal replacement therapies and drug treatments are negotiated, and how, in this process, the presence of the state is made real. Within these encounters, I concentrate on the various forms of paper-work that mediate these interactions, and which serve to materially demonstrate the contingent and arbitrary character of care (I would like this hyphenated formulation "paper-work" to incorporate an understanding of the array of documents that collectively embody and shape medical work as well as the work that needs to be expended in order for these documents to translate into forms of care. I will, therefore, refer to "paper-work" in relation to my ethnographic study, but will retain the use of "paperwork" when referring to the work of others).[2] As Akhil Gupta shows in his work on bureaucracy in India, readymade accounts of structural violence provide incomplete explanations for the violence of poverty. Poor people suffer despite their inclusion and importance to democratic politics and processes in India. In other words, the state is far from indifferent to the plight of poverty. Officials show concern; they want to help. Nonetheless, the practical bases upon which entitlements are determined through these encounters are contingent, even capricious, and lead to widely varying results for people. Orienting to these empirical practices rather than abstract formal accounts of what bureaucracies are expected to do thus avoids, in Gupta's terms, the trap of conflating the spectacle of disciplinary power with its operation. By examining the practical modalities through which harm and violence is exercised—even if not necessarily explicitly intended—within specific sites of governmental practice, Gupta illustrates that agents of the state do not have to be callous or charged with disciplinary zeal for their work to have such an effect, for their actions to violate everyday life and sociality and produce arbitrary outcomes. In essence, rather than look at the character of people, Gupta highlights the importance of looking at the nature of the practices in which they are engaged and how these practices shape outcomes. For Gupta, the point is "that such arbitrariness is not itself arbitrary; rather, it is systematically produced by the very mechanisms that are meant to ameliorate social suffering" (2012, 23).

Arbitrariness, contingency and the ambivalences inherent in state work are fundamental to the sites and interactions which shape the practice of renal care and, from there, people's highly unequal and differentiated access to it. Drawing on clinical consultations, with reference to anthropological work on the cultural life of the bureaucratic document (Goody 1968; Hull 2012b), I explore the kinds of scripts, prescriptions, letters of support, and so on that are produced within clinical encounters, and the multiple readings and forms of interpretation they are open to. These highly contingent and unstable cultural objects are not simply read, but are acted on in ways that are rarely easy to predict in advance. Patients, for example, petition doctors to produce *résumés* for them. These are legitimating scripts, which patients must have when attempting to access support and broker healthcare across public, private, and charitable domains. Doctors also informally manipulate prescriptions for medications to facilitate access to those whose costs are not covered by the state, or they will increase prescription quantities so that those enrolled in forms of insurance can share with those without. These localized, hidden, and contingent arrangements underpin the vulnerability of care for patients, while keeping them and their families continually "on the move" (as discussed in previous chapters). Importantly they also show doctors' practices to be highly circumscribed. As a result, we see institutional actors such as doctors emerge as equivocal and ambivalent agents of the state and market, who simultaneously embody and subvert the operations of both in the course of their everyday work.

THE CLINICAL ENCOUNTER

The interactions between health professionals (associated clinical specialists, nursing staff, nutritionists, social workers, pharmacists, psychologists, and laboratory technicians, among others) and kidney patients at all stages of their illness trajectories, are manifold and conducted across a wide range of clinical and extra-clinical spaces: in outpatient clinical consultations; in emergency rooms; during ward visits; in the homes of patients on CAPD; in hospital corridors, stairwells, and waiting rooms; and in the various public spaces and streets adjacent to the hospital.

Throughout my research, many queries and problems were resolved, and much work was accomplished, in these mundane interactions and spaces. Doctors were continually being interrupted by colleagues, and patients and phone calls would routinely delay meetings or consultations. A constant possibility, I never saw anyone refuse to respond to these ad hoc intrusions and say that they were too busy or in a hurry. Interruptions, grabbing a favorable moment when people are physically present, were simply part of how hospital work got done, one which turned happenstance into opportunity. Private or professional time, therefore, was far from privileged, and yet, no impression was given that the activities of doctoring were unduly pressured. Still, it often took me by surprise when doctors would say at the end of busy and congested consultation hours, "Ah, we have finished early." How exactly finishing early was achieved, or what signified that it had been, was never readily apparent.

Although many clinical encounters were spontaneous, this did not necessarily imply a lack of coherence or organization. In almost all cases, these encounters were fitted to the everyday demands of hospital life by the various types of paper-work that mediated them. Patient files, the daily patient census, scripts for prescribed medication, x-rays, ultrasounds, pathology requests, sets of dietary instructions, instructions to assist compliance, maps, résumés (referral letters or letters of introduction), and so on, grounded the interactions between doctors and patients and circulated throughout the hospital and beyond. This paper-work was critical as it joined up one set of clinical encounters with another and helped constitute patient trajectories of care and support. Paper-work could be seen less as a factual or bureaucratic documentation of sickness and its treatments, than a cultural resource to be drawn on in a variety of ways, depending on circumstances, to keep both patients and the work of medicine moving along.

In the ethnographic accounts that follow, I focus, for the most part, on the clinical consultation and the paper-work that was both productive of it and produced by it. That includes the list of documents above, yet this is by no means comprehensive, and the documents themselves are not records of all the situationally relevant facts, but instead stand testament to the contingent character of the doctor-patient relationship and its production of systemically arbitrary effects.

NEPHROLOGY WORK: THE DAILY ROUND

Ethnographic research in the hospital meant following the routines of nephrologists, in particular, the work of Ana and her team. Ana arrived at the hospital around 7:30 A.M. each morning to conduct ward rounds, as well as hold both pre-arranged and impromptu meetings with staff and patients. Afterward she would make her way to the *consultorios* (outpatient consultation rooms). She rarely got to them before 10 A.M., but continued until the last patient was seen, often around 1 P.M., leaving to return home a little after 2 P.M.

Her working day was not representative of those of her colleagues: she was one of the few doctors who did not hold multiple positions in the healthcare system. However, like other medical staff, she started her working day by printing out the daily "census" of patients from the only networked computer available on the fifth floor. This census—an Excel spread sheet, continually updated—provided details on the in-patients under the care of nephrology on any given day. On my first day following her through her routines, there were fifty-five patients recorded, all at different stages of treatment and kidney function. The census contained their names, ages, registration numbers, dates of admission, and their renal status (i.e., whether they were on dialysis or recovering from transplant surgery), pending treatments, and test results. Kidney donor details were also recorded here.

Although the census provided a structure to morning rounds, helping the doctors identify who needed to be seen and when, it was also offered as a tool to structure our ethnographic work, a practical mechanism for deciding which patients might be important for me to meet as well as amenable to interview. Ana would, therefore, ensure she had two printouts, one for her work and one for ours. In the early stages of research, the census—as a collection of dates, numbers, and biological measurements—was not always a clear guide for identifying ethnographic research participants. The only solution was to learn from Ana which patients presented particular concerns for her and why, and to proceed on that basis. One particular morning, she was keen to draw attention to six post-transplant patients all in hospital with complications, primarily infections and organ rejections. She explained that many of her patients contracted hospital-based infections and stressed that this meant their families would be faced with the additional costs of the antibiotics used to treat these infections, as they were with everything else. The dominant subject of our conversations was the challenges her patients faced as they progressed through different aspects of their healthcare.

The census, as suggested, is a daily and ephemeral survey of lying-in CKD patients. Yet, it was much less a mechanism for producing statistical information than an organizational device or means of coordinating the collective work of renal care. What is more, the information it contained was not always accurate, as we learned when presented with patients who were much younger or older than recorded on the census or whose kidney functioning was quantitatively better or worse than described. It was also an uncertain research tool for medical staff hoping to publish research papers based on their clinical work in the hospital. This we learned when Dr. Miguel Ángel, a young resident under Ana's supervision, attempted to use the census as a tracking device to identify patients who had failed to show up for planned treatments or appointments. In 2012 alone, out of one hundred patients registered with the hospital, thirty did not return. They had apparently gone missing.

Miguel Ángel wanted to investigate and initiated a study to find out why: to understand if they had moved, changed doctor or health provider, had died, or indeed had given up on the various efforts (moral, physical, or financial) required for their renal care. Using the census and the patient files linked to it, and so with a list of names, addresses, and the ages of patients, Cesar and I accompanied the young doctor as he drove around the city and its outskirts knocking on doors in an attempt to track down these missing patients. This proved to be an unrewarding task, particularly when addresses had only been partially entered or names misspelled or when, in some of the poorer barrios, it proved impossible to identify street names. Discussions with neighbors only sometimes yielded information. We did learn that one patient, Luisa Martinez had died, having spoken briefly to her granddaughter; that Jose Mercado wasn't missing at all but had recently showed up at clinical consultations; that Estela Garcia was on hemodialysis at IMSS. But in most cases, either the patient or the street they lived on could not be found. The census proved a better guide to the organizational setting within the hospital than anything outside it.

In many respects, the census invited us to ask what paper-work is and does, what it can help us to see and what it can make invisible. The ubiquity of documents of this kind—part of the mundane technologies of healthcare—is, as Matthew Hull (2012b) reminds us, easy to overlook and take for granted, particularly as the routine production of paper appears to give us immediate access to the very thing it documents. However, if we accept that bureaucratic paper-work are materials mediating social relations rather than offering unproblematic descriptions of them, then the visibilities such documents rely on and allow for can be examined. In the words of Latour, these materials "transform, translate, distort, and modify the meaning or the elements they are supposed to carry" (Latour in Hull 2012a: 253). The *consultorio* provided an extremely valuable site from which to observe the production of paper-work and the ways in which it shaped the care of kidney patients.

Consultorios

During fieldwork, consultations with outpatients were undertaken in temporary accommodation due to the construction of a new outpatients' wing. Situated next to this building site, the *consultorios* interim home was a set of prefabricated rooms connected by a long corridor that broke out into separate consultation spaces, many double units. There was space for twenty-three clinical consultations to take place at any one time. All were equipped with desks, two or three chairs, a small sink, and, in some of the slightly larger ones, a bed. None afforded much privacy for either patient or doctor. In the mornings, they were particularly over-crowded, and despite a system of timetabling, many medical specialists simply had to wait until space became available or find an alternative. Nephrology, nominally, had two rooms toward the end of the corridor.

Squeezed in between these rooms was a nurse's table piled high with boxes of assorted *carpetas* (folders containing patient files) and the *tarjeta de citas* (the appointment book). The corridor was a workspace used by teams of nurses and nutritionists preparing patients, recording information, and taking measurements. Meanwhile, patients and their families stood along the corridor, spilling out into an outdoor waiting area. They gathered from early morning until mid-afternoon, some with and some without appointments (see figure 5). A clinical timetable suggested that CAPD patients were seen before 10 A.M., transplant patients or patients preparing for a transplant between 10 A.M. and noon, and new patients in the afternoon. However, this never seemed to bear out in practice.[3] Rather, who got to be seen and when was not always a matter of organization and planning, of waiting one's turn. Instead, flexibility was built in; doctors asked favors for their own patients to be seen in clinically urgent cases and patients routinely popped in with the odd *pregunta* (question) or request for a résumé in the spaces between consultations.

One morning, Ana and I were sitting behind the consultation desk chatting. A woman popped her head in through the doorway and interrupted, *"Por favor . . . could the doctora advise?"* She was clearly distressed and wanted to talk about her son, a CAPD patient who had just been taken to the emergency room. He had peritoneal tuberculosis, an infection that Ana explained is easily disguised and hard to diagnose.[4] The son, in his early twenties, was in a serious condition. Previously he had had half of his colon removed and was reliant on a colostomy bag. His mother explained he had been eating tacos, after which he became very sick, and he was now facing a long hospital stay. He was losing a lot of fluid and his creatinine levels were very high.[5] His mother explained that she was her son's main carer and that looking after him was now her full-time occupation as she had recently lost her job in a gasoline station. The doctors wanted to do a biopsy but she could not afford the biopsy needles. She was also told that her son needed to take valganciclovir, a drug that cost roughly 22,000 pesos (1,764 U.S. dollars) a month.[6] She needed a six-month supply but only had enough for five months and now had to appeal for money and support from different charitable organizations.

What she wanted from Ana was a résumé—a letter of introduction from her as a nephrologist, which would explain her son's condition and her personal circumstances, and thereby legitimize her search for help and support. Ana smiled

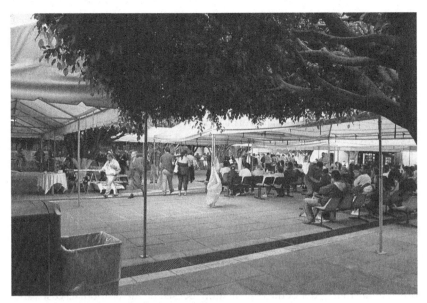

FIGURE 5. Waiting for medical appointments.

and said she was happy to provide the letter and support the woman's efforts. After exchanging a little further information, Ana told her when the letter would be ready and the woman, grateful, left. Ana explained that she and many of the other doctors spend a great deal of time, especially at the end of their shifts, writing résumés to help their patients get support for healthcare. "This is why," she stated, "we all carry our lap-tops around with us, so that we can do this wherever we are. Besides, there is only one computer in the residents' room."

The very next day when I returned to the consultorios, Ana was not there but had left a message with one of the nurses that I was to be accommodated. I was ushered in behind the desk of Dr. Miguel Ángel and Dr. Isabel, a younger trainee nephrologist. They were already in the middle of a consultation. Miguel Ángel nodded and smiled that it was fine for me to join them, but unlike Ana who went out of her way to make me comfortable, I had no idea how he felt about having to factor me into his morning routines and how much of a disruption I would be to his work. The only other chair available was used by Isabel and though I insisted I was happy to stand, a nurse was called to find another one. This, in effect, meant that three of us were now crammed in behind the small desk that faced the Hernandez family, whose consultation had been interrupted by my arrival.

The Hernandez family consisted of Alejandra, a sixteen-year-old kidney patient, and her mother. They had come to talk through the results of a biopsy and an x-ray, among other tests. Alejandra sat on the only chair positioned on her side of the table, while her mother stood beside her, asking questions. At different points in the conversation, the doctors talked between themselves while mother and daughter listened patiently. Miguel Ángel wanted to know how Alejandra had been getting on over the course of the past year.

Despite my proximity, I was finding it hard to hear the conversation amid the sound of drilling outside the makeshift consultorios and the constant flow of people coming in and out through the open door. I did learn that Alejandra's kidneys were still working at 50 percent of their original functioning and that as a result, she was not yet on any form of dialysis. At the same time, there had been an increase of protein in her urine, and the doctors were concerned that this was only set to worsen. Miguel Ángel, in an effort to reassure mother and daughter, talked through a set of statistics to explain how well and for how long patients can live with limited renal functioning as long as, that is, they looked after their diet.

The cause of Alejandra's kidney failure was glomerulonephritis.[7] She also had two brothers with CKD, which prompted Isabel to emphasize the importance of having a clinical family history done. With that, she wrote a referral letter for Alejandra to see someone in the medical school at the University of Guadalajara. Much of the remainder of the consultation focused on medication, its costs, and whether the type of medical insurance the Hernandez family had would cover it. Alejandra's mother explained they had Seguro Popular, and they already knew that it would not support most of the medications her daughter would need. Just as the consultation drew to a close, there was a small pause, after which Alejandra's mother asked if Miguel Ángel could write a résumé as she would need to find financial support to pay for the prescriptions he was writing. He agreed to do so and they left.

Requests for résumés were a central feature of clinical consultations, and I did not hear any request made turned down. This short letter of introduction, detailing the clinical case and needs of the patient, in so many respects, materialized patient trajectories of care as well as symbolized the contingencies that accessing care rested on. These modes of inscription kept patients legitimately on the move, opening up new channels for medical care and support as they did. Although such requests were an informal part of the clinical consultation—dependent on the needs of patients and their families, as well as their willingness to ask—they were, nevertheless, a culturalized means of dealing with the limitations of healthcare provision—limitations that constrained the work of doctors as well as the well-being and recovery of patients.

Résumés were far from "hidden transcripts" in James Scott's (1990) use of the term; they were not favors, nor acts of subterfuge to counteract the work of more dominant forces, but locally workable ways of doing healthcare. However, because the outcomes of providing résumés could never be specified or guaranteed in advance, this meant that extraordinary levels of arbitrariness were bound up with the "social life" of these documents. This arbitrariness adversely affected the health and lives of patients and their families, who could do little more than follow where their documents would take them, and then deal with what they found once there. This often necessitated further movement backed by further documentation.

The normalization and banality of locally workable practices are key to understanding the various ways in which harms are inflicted on Mexico's poorer citizens by state institutions like health and welfare (Livingstone 2012). At the same time, most of the doctors I observed acted out of care, with many going far beyond what was required of them in terms of their daily duties to provide support to their patients. Their status, as doctors, was ambivalent. On one hand, they were fellow citizens eager to find ways of working around the restrictions patients encountered; on the other, they were agents of the state, implicated in setting patients and their families on haphazard routes to create their own regimes of renal care.

Patient Files

Almost immediately after Alejandra left, Andrea Flores walked in with her mother and father. She sat down, and her parents stood behind her. Her mother directed the discussion, armed with questions, each one graphically illustrated by her daughter's many test results, prescriptions, and x-rays, all passed over to Miguel Ángel, one by one, by Andrea's father. Isabel checked the scripts, making a note that Andrea was taking steroids, prednisone, cortisone, and aspirin and didn't seem to have experienced any problems or side effects. Her mother questioned the quantity of pills her daughter was taking and wanted some of her test results explained. Isabel responded but her explanations were rapid and without any translation of clinical terms. Both doctors went through the paperwork discussing the respective and changing statuses of the patient's proteinuria and creatinine, both important diagnostic indicators of kidney function.

Miguel Ángel's phone rang and he left the room for about ten minutes. While he was gone, Isabel asked the father for an x-ray result and started to examine it. She held it up to the light for almost four minutes, without saying anything, then read the accompanying letter, again taking her time, but without saying anything. As the parents watched her patiently, she moved from x-ray to letter and back again. She turned to me to talk about the presence of protein in the urine and explained that they were looking for an infection but there wasn't one. Andrea had been diagnosed a year ago with CKD and had been relatively stable, but there was now clear evidence of a further decrease in kidney functioning. Isabel explained, again to me, that they would need to increase some of her medications, and with that Miguel Ángel returned to squeeze past me. I felt acutely that I was an intrusion.

Miguel Ángel sat back down, saying *mira* (look), as a way to arrest attention and refocus discussion. He explained the results slowly to the family, letting them know there was a deterioration in Andrea's condition, while smiling and looking at all of them, in turn, as he spoke. He discussed Andrea's diet and stressed the need for the family to be very strict. Andrea's mother explained that her daughter ate little fat, but mostly fish, chicken, and cereals. Miguel Ángel simply reasserted his point and repeated what she could and could not eat.

He then looked at the results of a pelvic exam and the accompanying letter in silence. The mother finally asked if it was normal. Miguel Ángel said yes, and then outlined the challenges of having CKD for a girl of Andrea's age when his phone rang again. This happened four more times during the consultation. After each interruption he apologized, reengaging the family's attention with *mira*, holding up another piece of paper, while emphasizing how critical it was for the family to comply with the treatment regime. They went on to discuss a small rash of spots that had recently appeared on Andrea's upper arms, face, and lower neck as well as some light bruising on her cheek. Miguel Ángel talked through her medications, writing further prescriptions but also sets of instructions that explained how and when to take them. He copied some of the information from Andrea's test results into a patient file, when his phone rang for a final time and he handed back all of the paper-work to the family for them to resume responsibility.

This accumulation of paper-work comprises an extensive mobile archive, generating the most comprehensive body of documentation on the uncertain trajectories patients and their families take to access renal services in Mexico. Added to in every encounter, gaining layers and more bulk depending on the complexity of each case, this mobile archive shows how information moves between patients and medical specialties, different clinics, and sites of support. That this archive is maintained by the family rather than any sited health provider teaches us a great deal about how the moral economy of healthcare is organized and the pivotal role of families within it.

Paper-work proliferates during the clinical encounter as more drug prescriptions, test results, instructions, notes, and patient files are written for inclusion within it. Taken together, they provide the material ground of explanation, requests, and reassurances, as well as rearticulations of the demands for compliance and the delivery of bad news. For the patient and their family, they become guides to further action. Acquiring paperwork also necessitates acts of deference, as well as learning the language, gestures, and performances expected within the clinical encounter. To return briefly to James Scott (1990), these documents produce a type of "public transcript," which require patients to learn the established ways of behaving and speaking necessary to the clinical encounter.[8] They are an expression of the conformity expected of patients when under medical care and serve to routinize and normalize everyday clinical practice and action.

Instructions and Prescriptions

My next opportunity to shadow Ana was a week later. I was hoping that we would have an opportunity to talk, as I wanted to check my understanding of the previous week's consultations. I woke early that morning to a storm, typical for August in Guadalajara. It had been raining since the very early hours. I had been optimistic it would stop before I left for the hospital, as was generally the case, but it didn't. The rain got heavier and I had to call for a taxi. By the time I arrived at the hospital, I stepped out into a river of rainwater flowing through the streets around the hospital, and was immediately soaked through. Even inside the hospital, the rain continued to come down with great force, producing waterfalls throughout the old colonnades. The rain made its way into the waiting areas for patients, which were by 8:45 A.M. completely full.

Walking through the hospital corridors, the electricity flickered on and off before it cut out completely. The hospital's ageing electrical generators then ground into action and the corridor lights slowly made their way back on. I felt tired and wet but could not begin to imagine how staff or patients adjusted to the unpredictable, though not unusual, conditions that are part of the Jaliscan rainy season. As the weather affects many of the staff coming to work, services often have to be suspended. Because of the storm, the hospital elevators were out of order and I walked up the narrow staircase, past the broken toilets, to the fifth floor, and let myself into the residents' room with the key Ana had provided so we could have a work space whenever we were in the hospital. This freedom to come and go was never lost on me.

Almost immediately, patients popped their heads around the doorway to look for Ana. I could hear her talking to some pharmaceutical representatives further down the corridor. She eventually made her way into the room with a woman who wanted to talk through her protocol for living-related organ donation. The woman was thirty-four-year-old Josefina, the mother and potential organ donor for her seventeen-year-old son, Felipe. Josefina was carrying a large pink and blue striped shopping bag; inside it was a bulky plastic folder with her son's medical notes, prescription scripts, test results, and so on.

The conversation focused primarily on what they needed to do to prepare for the surgery and the importance of both mother and son maintaining a good diet. Ana took out a book that she particularly liked to use with patients, one that I'd seen her draw on many times in consultations, *Dieta Para Estar en La Zona* (*The Zone Diet* by Barry Sears). They talked through the book's core message, while Ana wrote a number of scripts for medications and a series of dietary instructions. Josefina wanted to know if Seguro Popular would cover her prescription costs and Ana explained that it did so only in some cases. Ana continued to write, explaining in detail which medications were covered by Seguro Popular and which ones were not, but she also explained that she would do her best to write the prescriptions in such a way as to mask the underlying CKD. When she finished writing, she turned to me in English saying, "sometimes, we need to lie; if we don't, they [Seguro Popular] won't cover the costs." This often meant emphasizing CKD-related conditions that are covered by Seguro Popular, such as hypertension, without mentioning CKD itself. Manipulating prescriptions in this way was a further strategy to make up for systematic limitations of the system. Like so many of the other forms of improvisation that are part of the work of doctoring and treating CKD in Mexico, they created little by way of stability or predictability for patients.

Josefina, assertive throughout, asked lots of questions. After almost thirty minutes, she left and Maricela, the social worker linked to the hemodialysis unit, popped her head in. Ana took the opportunity to fix a time for Cesar and me to interview her and learn more about her work. After Maricela left, there was another patient waiting, hoping to get Ana's attention, and I realized that I would not get to talk to her that day.

The residents' room where we were sitting was not a private working space, but somewhere for the doctors to sit, catch up on bits of paper-work or have conversations with patients and each other. It was adjacent to another staff room, usually occupied by young trainee doctors and nurses, and where the census was printed out each morning. The residents' room was small, about ten feet by fourteen feet. It had a table and eight chairs, which filled the room to capacity, although I never saw it full. Against one wall was a water cooler, an old computer, and a large fan. Against the other wall stood a filing cabinet and a cupboard haphazardly stuffed with random documents, old computer cables, and a large brown box full of patient files. I later discovered that this brown box contained copies of patient protocols for living-related kidney donations. That day, the room was incredibly warm. Due to the storm, the electricity supply had not resumed functioning in all parts of the hospital, which meant that the fan did not work and there was no release from the heat.

Among many other passers-by, Maria, one of the renal nurses, entered the room with a phone call for Ana, followed by Gloria, the mother and organ donor of Carlos, whom we met in the introduction. Gloria was looking for prescriptions for antibiotics and immunosuppressants. Ana sat down to write Gloria's scripts and then a series of instructions, numbered one to ten, which explained in great detail how to take these particular medications. Compliance with medications, for post-transplant patients, is critical, and so medical staff instruct patients' consumption as thoroughly as they can. Instructions, however, are provided in the absence of understanding the specific and contextual difficulties any given patient may have in taking medications regularly, such as literacy, deciphering handwriting, poverty, and the pressures of everyday living, the varying associations patients make between taking medication and feeling sick, or simply not wanting to. Instructions materialize the insistences of compliance, of doing whatever one is told to do whether one likes it or not. They are written with anticipated contingencies in mind but they are not negotiable—a flexible inflexibility.

After spending some time in the residents' room, Ana and I made our way down to the *consultorios*, where the hallways were packed to capacity. Seated in one of the double-consultation rooms was Teresa Gonzalez, a young woman of twenty-two, who had come in with her mother. The mother pointed to the dark circles around her daughter's eyes, while Ana asked her to see her tongue and her nails. Teresa was on her second deceased-donor transplant and had come to Hospital Civil via IMSS where her transplant surgery had been carried out.

Ana was concerned that Teresa was not looking after her diet and asked one of the nutritionists to come in to talk through a *plan de alimentation* (a food or nutrition plan), and to draw up a list of what foods Teresa could and could not have. Ana explained that Teresa had been given similar plans and instructions many times before but that it was important to keep reinforcing the message. She looked through Teresa's most recent test results and transferred them to a large hospital *carpeta* (file). I asked how this information would be managed and stored. Ana said that the nephrology team looked after their own patient files, adding that if they were sent to a centralized office, it would be months before they would see their patients again. For similar reasons, she and her colleagues made their own *citas* (appointments) with patients. She showed me her work diary, a little note book on which she had glued a picture of two kidneys, which was full of patient information and appointment times and dates. This information, she said, was in duplicate and managed by the renal nurses so that they could make whatever arrangements they needed to locally.

Another family arrived just as this encounter ended. Thomas, who was eighty-five, stepped into the consultation room with his son and daughter. The son told Ana his father couldn't hear well, and he spoke on his behalf. Thomas sat on a chair holding onto his cane and exchanged glances with me and Ana. He was a category-four renal patient, meaning that his kidney failure was rapidly advancing, but had not yet reached end stage. While a nurse took Thomas's blood pressure, Ana checked his most recent test results, making calculations based on his filtration rates and creatinine levels as she did so. Thomas said he had vomited after eating, that he had a lot of stomach acid, and that he was often very hungry. He assured Ana that he had been taking his pills, and with that, his daughter handed over a list of his medications, reiterating the point about vomiting as she did.

Ana asked about his eyes, but Thomas referred to his hands and feet instead and explained that they were swollen. Ana smiled and reached across the desk to hand him a piece of paper, saying slowly that he was only to take a quarter of the medication written down. Thomas was concerned about his sleep, particularly as he experienced many of his symptoms at night. The conversation continued on the subject of medication, the quantities that had to be taken and the intervals they had to be taken at, quickly followed by a discussion about the limits of Seguro Popular, the family's medical costs, and their difficulties in meeting them.

The family wanted to know about opportunities for dialysis, given how advanced Thomas's condition was, but Ana told them it was unlikely to be an option. Thomas was old and dialysis would put untold pressure both on him and his family. Her preference was that his condition be managed through diet and medication. Ana wrote down everything she had said, distilling her core messages into eight points and then discussing each one in turn, twice. Thomas's daughter checked through all the information, questioning Ana's handwriting here and there. Ana took out her smart phone and looked for the phone number of a nutritionist who could help them further, after which Thomas's son went through her instructions one more time for clarification.

Clarification is equally important for both medical staff and patients in these encounters. In the moves made between different institutions and systems of care, mistakes frequently occur. If tests, for instance, have to be re-run, patients and their families incur additional expenses and treatment schedules are interrupted, affecting medical work as well as the health and wellbeing of patients.

Errors

On occasion, we went to the *consultorios* in the afternoon to observe Dr. Fernando, another consultant nephrologist. The consultation rooms were much quieter in the afternoons and Fernando had no difficulty finding a space to work. His first appointment was with seventeen-year-old Daniel, who arrived with his mother. They brought with them a series of laboratory test results and wanted to talk through some blood tests and Daniel's creatinine levels. Daniel, a cancer patient with declining kidney function, needed a second opinion due to confusion over the precise nature of his renal diagnosis.

Approximately fifteen months before, Daniel had had an appointment with Ana, who identified problems with kidney functioning and told him he would need a biopsy. She also mentioned that he was dehydrated. He was given a follow-up appointment, but the doctor he saw next contradicted Ana's judgement, telling him he did not need a biopsy and to continue with his medication regime, but that he should be monitored monthly. At one of these monthly appointments, another doctor told him he did need a biopsy because there was an increase of protein in his urine. As Daniel also had leukemia and was undergoing chemotherapy, in addition to receiving conflicting advice, his mother delayed proceeding with the matter further. She was concerned he would be given more medication that might affect his blood pressure and she didn't want to damage his heart.

A family friend encouraged her to seek further opinion, saying that she knew the director of Hospital Civil and was greatly impressed by the reputation of doctors there. They were referred to Fernando, who requested preliminary tests before having a biopsy; it was these results they were to discuss. In addition to a routine testing of kidney functioning, Fernando requested hepatitis C and B and a HIV test to ensure there were no interfering conditions. On reading through the results, he commented, "they didn't do the hep C exams? I don't know why the lab didn't do them because I always request these three together. I am going to call them to see what happened." He immediately called the lab, explaining that he sent a patient down for three tests but only two had been returned. The lab technician assured him that all the tests had been done, but only two had been filled in on the paperwork due to an oversight. Fernando said he would have to send the patient back to pick up the outstanding results.

Fernando told Daniel he was aware that he had been given confusing information and reassured him that he would explore the matter further. However, Daniel would now have to have a biopsy and an appointment needed to be made sooner rather than later. He cautioned that hospital services were saturated:

> If we tell you to come tomorrow, it is possible that we won't have a bed and will have to give you another date. If we can get a bed, that will be good, and it might be the case that we can do the biopsy that day. But remember you will need to bring the needle for the biopsy. Dr. Martín, who you will see next, will tell you what kind you need, how much it will cost and where to buy it as well as how much you will pay when you take the biopsy to the pathology lab.

Directly after Daniel left, Jorge, another doctor in the hospital, came in to look for a favor for his son who was very ill. His son's protein levels were particularly high and so he had arranged for a specialist to conduct tests. He had received the results but wanted to discuss them with Fernando. As they read through the paperwork together, Fernando exclaimed, "you requested a lot of exams—your son's blood count shows anemia, the urea is high, the cholesterol and triglycerides are high and the protein also high. He should also have had a 24 hour urine test. Where is it?" His friend suggested the specialist may not have done this.

Fernando confirmed that Jorge's son's kidneys were small and there was evidence of chronic damage. However, the kidneys were functioning, and Fernando explained that if treated properly, they could maintain this level of functioning for some years. However, it was necessary to conduct the urine tests. He continued, "we don't need to do this here, in fact, we often don't request them here because they don't do it properly, so you can go wherever you want—go to a lab you trust, perhaps a private clinic that you prefer and then we can meet again."

What we learn about the type of paper-work that mediates the clinical encounter is that it does not produce a straightforward or reliable account of diagnostic processes. Paper-work, instead, can be read as a methodological issue—not just for the ethnographer—but for the clinical practitioner also. Despite the persistence of errors on various documents, they are, nonetheless, navigationally significant, providing sets of coordinates from which it is possible to see where patients have been and from there what might need to be done to prepare them for where they have to go next. Paper-work suggests little can be taken for granted by doctors or patients. Paper-work thus provides waymarks and makes it possible to see the joins between different arenas of healthcare activity. Operating at various points between different levels and layers of medical work, using such documentation can be as complex for medical staff as it is for the medically untrained, only serving to underline the arbitrary and contingent character of care and its organization for both. Nonetheless, clinical paper-work helps to reconstruct the "logic of care" as a situated and locally defined practice (Mol 2008).

CRAFTING A MORAL ECONOMY OF CARE

Reflecting on the subject of bureaucratic paperwork, Gupta explains:

> Writing functions to note, to record, and to report. However, it would be a mistake to see writing as that which follows action. It is not as if officials first conduct meetings, discussions, inspections, observations, and surveys and then write down what transpires in the course of those actions. Rather, writing itself needs to be seen as the central activity of bureaucracies. Writing precedes, accompanies and follows other actions. It does not merely record what happened but is the main activity that takes place in bureaucratic work. (2012, 149)

And so, by extension, while patient files, prescriptions, instructions, letters of introduction, and so on invite a descriptive reading, these various documents need to be read in relation to the exigencies of the given situations and everyday understandings in which they are embedded. They cannot be read literally or taken at face value, whatever that might mean. Perhaps they function best as moral documents, responding and reflecting what is at stake for others, embodying the entangled sets of relationships and the rights and obligations that are situationally an element of those relations. Paperwork, fundamental to the clinical encounter, is not just a by-product. Far from it: it plays a constitutive role. Because it is constitutive, paperwork teaches us much about the arbitrary and contingent character of access to healthcare. Gupta contends such contingency is harmful in its effects, not because it *is* contingent or arbitrary, but because such contingencies are systematically produced and normalized in ways that institutionalize harm.

Paperwork keeps things moving, a function which Crowley-Matoka (2016) noted too in her ethnographic work on transplant medicine in Mexico. She emphasizes the significance and use of the verb *agilizar* within Mexican clinical encounters. *Agilizar* means to move things along; to move through the bureaucratic system of health care; to leverage social relationships. By way of example, she describes Arturo, who was desperately seeking access to the transplant program at the Ministry for Health.

> Giving up on the official channels, Arturo drew on his extended family network to cobble together the money for bus fare and came to Guadalajara on his own, where he showed up in person on the transplant floor. Dressed in clothes both conspicuously worn and spotlessly clean, he bore carefully organized copies of his complete medical chart from his local clinic. Polite, friendly and persistent, Arturo was indefatigably patient as he waited around the program floor for hours at a time

over a several-day period, telling and retelling his story to various people. Each time he was told that he needed a referral from his local doctor for admittance into the program, he would nod his head in understanding, then inquire with gentle insistence if, after all, there weren't some other way to move things along, some other person he might be able to speak with to plead his case. Staff began to note his persistence and level of motivation to one another in tones of nearly equal irritation and admiration, and eventually his strategic self-presentation and resolve paid off. Circumventing the usual referral requirements, arrangements were made by one of the staff nephrologists to admit him directly into the transplant program for evaluation. (Crowley-Matoka 2016, 122)

Arturo is like the many patients I have encountered who come to medical consultations armed with their medical files, records, and test results, looking for ways and means to progress next steps. Essential as paper-work is in facilitating, extending, and multiplying clinical encounters, most of it, however, never acquires bureaucratic or organizational stability or permanence. That paper-work is as mobile as the patient and their family is an acknowledged effect of poor record keeping within clinical settings. Critically important as it is to both patient and doctor, this paper-work does not leave a formal trace (Bowker and Star 1999). It does not produce a public history.

In many respects, the means-to-end mode of record-keeping and its role in linking together healthcare regimes and infrastructures stands in sharp contrast to the formal account of healthcare access grounded in social entitlement and welfare arrangements, described in chapters 2 and 3. These arrangements appear to belong to a world defined by bureaucratic rationalities, but those rationalities fail to translate into everyday practice. Mobile archives of paper, and the social relations in which they are embedded and to which they give rise, orient patients and their families to a moral economy of care where they and not the state or any other sited provider must take responsibility.[9] Borrowing from Nading (2017), paperwork "crafts" this moral economy.[10] It keeps families on the move and materializes their responsibilities for others. It grounds the clinical encounter in shared but unregistered understandings. As Nading suggests, it works to "close the distance" between patients and healthcare professionals as collaborators and, at times, co-conspirators, in attempting to make healthcare work. It also serves to disguise and cover up the very problems that make strategic paperwork so critical in the first place. This is one of the dark ironies of the situation.

Matthew Hull (2012a) suggests that one of the reasons documents and paperwork have, until recently, been overlooked in anthropological research, is that paperwork elsewhere often appears to be so like our own. As a result, we can fail to recognize that what it means and does is significantly different from place to place, that it acquires its significance under very particular conditions. The paper-work

that travels with uninsured Mexican patients are some of the only material mani-
festations of their status as citizens, a status that other forms of bureaucratic work
(e.g., population health statistics and hospital-based patient records) have largely
left invisible. In this sense, paper-work is critical, both materially and methodologically (Riles 2006). Focusing on the empirical practices bound up with producing and acting on paper-work takes us beyond the totalizing frame of state
structures, to the arbitrariness, contingency, and ambivalences inherent in forms
of bureaucratic (structural) violence. In this way, paper-work "makes a world"
(Goodman 1978). The next chapter continues to emphasize the importance of
world-making practices, through the mechanisms of exchange, the extra-clinical
interfaces they inhabit, and the multiple forms they take to indigenize renal care
in Mexico.

5 · EXCHANGE

Bodies as Sites for the Production of (Surplus) Value

In late summer 2012, Agradecimiento A Familia y Personas Donadores—"A Day of Gratitude to Families and Those Who Have Donated"—was held in Guadalajara to acknowledge those who had gifted organs, both living and deceased. The event was a formal affair: one with wine and a buffet lunch; with a top table of dignitaries—surgeons, politicians, and bureaucrats; with gifts and promotional packs sponsored by pharma companies and charities; and with the imperative to promote and publicize organ donation. The occasion, organized around a series of talks by both donor families and recipients chosen to relay moving personal testimony before the invited audience, as well as a presentation ceremony with certificates of thanks for donors, started with a short film—*Por Siempre* (Forever) by film maker, Luis Felipe Ybarra Becker. It featured a father carrying his young injured son in his arms, moments after a car accident, his wife visibly distressed. They travel to a hospital, where the boy is rushed into surgery, but the doctors can't save him. The hospital is sanitized, private, and Americanized. The parents are middle class. Soon after the death of the young boy, organ donation is discussed, and decisions are made. The film ends with the funeral of the child. It provokes tears and upset among the attending families. It captures the grief and emotional distress that is inevitably bound to the gifting of an organ but is silent on the very nature of what giving means and requires practically and morally, particularly in a context where organs are predominantly given through living-related donation and not deceased donation. The extraordinary difficulties that attend the uncomplicated moral directive of this film—that gifting organs is materialized by the urge to do so, is noble and altruistic, and should be entered into when circumstances conspire to offer one the opportunity to act for the good of others—are an absent presence. The film tells us nothing about the complexities upon which organ transfer rests in Mexico, which ultimately demarcate the boundaries between who gives and who receives, and, moreover, between *what* is given and *what* is received.

The unpredictable lines of movement Mexican patients must take to secure support, as described in chapter 2 and the systemic, bureaucratic, and institutional arrangements that necessitate that movement, as discussed in chapters 3 and 4, mean that poor and sick bodies in search of organs for transplant draw around them all manner of events, processes, and interactions that embody radically different kinds of exchange between very different kinds of actor. In taking up the idea that failing kidneys establish transactions of many different kinds, this chapter draws on the well-established literature on organ exchange in anthropology, in particular on how the processes of gift-giving, commodification, and forms of reciprocity link together the social and the biological, the personal and the public, across both local and global terrains.

Rather than simply focus attention on organs as the sole subject of exchange, my purpose here is to broaden our thinking to include forms of exchange that are necessary for organ transplantation to occur. These include, as I've already stated, gifts solicited and unsolicited; conditional and unconditional forms of support; social transfers in the forms of benefits and social insurance pay-outs; and contractual obligations, barter, and monetary exchange, among other things. Extending across state, medical, and societal domains, instead of confined to any one of them, I show how kidney transplantation is both generative of and generated by such mutually intersecting forms of exchange, and is ultimately dependent on them. Specifically, I argue that those at the periphery of social welfare and entitlement in Mexico have little choice but to link together these modes of exchange and, in so doing, coproduce new markets in medicine.

ORGANS AS VALUE-PRODUCING ITEMS

Organs-for-transplant and the matrices of exchange on which they depend are key sites in the production of value(s), economically, biologically, and morally. These values are expressed in the measurable values of extending life years, the surplus value generated through expanding healthcare markets, the calculated attributions of value that emerge through the codification and equivalence work of tissue typing and antigen matching, and the moral values that extend from the complex configurations of care and responsibility that knit themselves across familial, institutional, and auxiliary sites and settings. Ultimately, organs-for-transplant are things of immense value, made so through the practices, processes, and discourses that show them to be scarce (Sharp 2006). The construction of organs as scarce and precious has driven their multiple modes of exchange as things to be gifted, bought and sold, stolen, and so on (Cohen 2002; Crowley-Matoka 2005, 2016; Hamdy 2012; Kierans 2015; Scheper-Hughes 2000). Their scarcity imbues them with politics (Bijker 2007).

Interactions between forms of value, bodily exchange, and technology have produced a substantial body of thinking on the issue of "biovalue" (Waldby and Mitchell 2006; Novas 2006) and its correlate "biocapital" (Sunder Rajan 2006; Rose 2007; Helmreich 2007). Not unlike biopolitics or bioeconomy, these neologisms show the body to be bound to a calculus of cost and benefit (Birch and Tyfield 2012). To avoid overdetermining the relationship of the body and its parts to market capitalism, or to assume notions of value as determinants of exchange, I examine how values are produced and reproduced by transplant medicine in emergent ways, by tracing their meanings outward to the unplanned places, contexts, and sites where they acquire relevance. By following uninsured CKD patients in their search for care, we understand how cultures of exchange—reciprocal, altruistic, market-based, compensatory, discursive, and so on—produce value. Furthermore, we see how the entangled character of these forms of exchange challenge the analytically fixed distinctions between organs as "gifts" versus "commodities."

FORMS OF GIVING: INTIMATE, FAMILIAL, AND LOCAL

I met Gabriel only weeks after his body rejected the kidney his mother had donated to him. The transplant surgery was achieved at great cost and both mother and son were now trying to come to terms with the cruel disappointment of having to return to the daily regimen of dialyzing at home. The youngest of seven children, Gabriel was diagnosed with CKD in 2008, four years prior to our meeting, and started on peritoneal dialysis soon after. His diagnosis coincided with his embarking on a master's degree in mathematics and oceanography, and although Gabriel had completed his studies, CKD had dismantled his hopes of a university career. It also meant that, unlike his siblings, he would not leave the family home he shared with his parents in a small village by Lake Chapala. Like many of the patients featured in this book, Gabriel didn't know why any of this had happened to him. He didn't know why he had CKD:

> I don't know what I can say. I was told I had *riñones chicos* [small kidneys] when I was diagnosed. When I was a small child, I don't think I looked after myself very well. At school I was diagnosed with encephalitis and given a lot of medication, maybe too many drugs and perhaps they were not good for my kidneys. When I found out I had CKD at university, this was really difficult . . . for all of us, particularly the cost of everything. We are not a family with money. My father is a waiter in a local restaurant, my mother is a housewife, nothing more, and I only had a small grant when studying, and that was that.

The emotional and financial burden that preparing for a kidney transplant entailed was made worse by its brevity. Gabriel felt that the organ rejected because he didn't take his immunosuppression medication properly. He explained that he wasn't provided with clear instructions how to do so, nor did he fully understand the significance of it. His mother, who sat beside, said, while crying, "I gave it [the kidney] to you, and it was all a tremendous expense. When we travelled to the hospital, there was no more money even to buy food. God must not have wanted you to have it."

Very soon after the kidney stopped working, Gabriel was offered another organ, this time from a deceased organ donor, but the family refused it. His mother explained that the doctors had even offered to delay the payments to facilitate the surgery:

> He [the doctor] said, come today, you can pay tomorrow, but I explained it isn't that easy. He said you need only 6,849 pesos [365 U.S. dollars] for the cross-match tests. I said, but we know how much everything *really* costs, so we said no, we will wait until we have the money. He said "are you going to waste the opportunity?" and we said, yes. A transplant . . . for everything . . . is somewhere between 67,000 and 82,000 pesos [3,600–4380 U.S. dollars]. Everything has to be bought, even the material for stitching the wound. It is too much for a family. . . . And Seguro Popular, we don't have it for all this. For us, it only covers consultations and one or two pills. Even the doctors complain about it. It doesn't make sense, there is no point in it. It's just a government lie.

There was little else for Gabriel to do but return to the daily routines of home dialysis. That he could do this at all was made possible by the good will and support of kin and community. His *cuarto de diálisis* (dialysis room) was made from plywood and assembled by the carpentry skills of a neighbor. It was made to fit within the already existing space of the family's living room. It blocked out a great deal of natural sunlight and significantly constrained family activities and gatherings. In sharp contrast to the clutter of everyday life around it, the room was painted white and kept free from personal items. It comprised a bed, a microwave for heating up dialysate solution, weighing scales, and countless boxes of dialysate solution, all sourced and stocked by the combined efforts and donations of family and friends (see figure 6). Only a crucifix and a handful of religious pictures pointed out to a realm beyond this para-clinical space.

The *cuarto de diálisis* dominated this small two-story house, the bottom floor of which was occupied by Gabriel's family and the upper floor by another family. Both families shared a small garden that sat at the entrance of the house, with a well-tended flowerbed in one corner and a guava tree heavy with fruit in the other. There was little separating the rooms inside; only curtains marked out their functional distinctions. Once inside, the ubiquitous boxes of dialysate solution were stacked from floor to ceiling in every available space in the living room as well as the

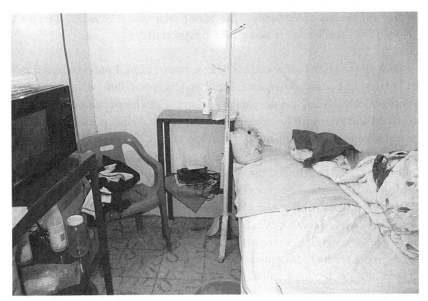

FIGURE 6. Gabriel's home dialysis room.

cuarto de diálisis, almost completely blocking an extensive collection of family photographs.

The boxes of dialysate solution had their own complex logistical life. Some were bought by money raised or borrowed from family, friends, and/or money lenders; others were sourced from local families via an informal distribution network that provided such things as dialysate solution, disinfectant, medications, and so on, particularly after loved ones were transplanted or had died. Others still were the outcome of negotiation with hospital social workers or procured from the new charitable and philanthropic bodies that had emerged in the context of a growing population of kidney patients across the state of Jalisco. Local, informal distribution networks were critical to families like Gabriel's, particularly those living at a distance from the city. Not only did they allow for the circulation of much needed medical items, these networks embodied their own wisdoms, histories of suffering, advice, and therapeutic value, and were generated and sustained by every day and enduring forms of sociality. Gabriel's mother explained:

> For *las aguas* [the waters, i.e., the dialysate solution], I dedicate myself to visiting. If I know they [other families with a CKD patient] have insurance and they have a water or two, then maybe I can share or borrow. I have to do this as there is often not even enough money to buy food. Gabriel is now just starting to work [having recently secured employment in a local technical college] and that feels good, but the income for a teacher in mathematics is not very high . . . So with the help of

God and the help of the family . . . we come forward and tell others that we can't pay in the hope they can do something to support us.

Dialysate solution is only one costly item among many. Routine hospital visits and tests are continually required. For laboratory tests, Gabriel relied on an aunt who ran a local clinical laboratory and who provided, for her nephew, medical tests on credit and at a much lower price than the hospital laboratories. While this provided something of a financial reprieve, costs still had to be repaid, and the necessity of doing so ensured the family was caught in a perpetual cycle of indebtedness.[1] Nevertheless, the pooling and circulation of medical supplies, made possible by the reciprocal character of local relationships, though offering no stability or sustainability, provided some solace for families like Gabriel's. In an echo of Polanyi's "stark utopia," where the increasing absences of adequate social investment and state support transfer the responsibilities of government from the public to the private realm, patients, without entitlement, become dependent on these contingent, localized, and ultimately fragile and easily overwhelmed sources of care.

These close, hand-to-hand forms of assistance organized around interpersonal interactions between networks of known contacts always threaten to degenerate into their own entropic spirals. They require huge investment on an ongoing basis if they are not to collapse. They thus multiply harm and risk. Moreover, they can only ever be supplementary to a much wider mixed economy of welfare and civil society forms. The question at the center of this book is how renal care reconfigures and depends on this mixed economy of welfare. As I go on to show, it carries its own sequential logics. Extending and facilitating access to renal care, in particular, transplant medicine produces its own effects and failings, particularly when more formalized and financialized arrangements of giving cannot possibly meet mechanisms that "grow demand." Paraphrasing Anna Tsing (2015), I ask, what kind of sociotechnical arrangement manages to survive, indeed thrive, in the ruins of welfare? What happens to renal care as it beds into a context of this particular kind?

THE BUREAUCRATIZATION OF GIVING-AS-CHARITY

Following the labor of patients like Gabriel inevitably leads to one of the many new charitable associations that have emerged to address the growing needs of kidney patients. In almost all cases, these associations have been established by patients or family members of patients, more often than not, middle-class families working in conjunction with senior healthcare professionals. The Association, as I will simply refer to it, was one such organization. Little more than a five-minute walk from the public hospital, it occupied a small two-story, leased house that could barely be seen from behind the large promotional banner stretching across its entire lower floor. Its main reception area was one story up, opening onto the side of a large tiled, multi-purpose room, and then on into a corporate style, though modestly furnished, meeting room. Toward the back of the room were toilets and a number of well-stocked store rooms neatly packed with medications and medical supplies, variously donated or bought at reduced price from pharmacies, pharmaceutical representatives, or families who no longer required them.

The Association was formally and legally constituted in 2009. It was formed by a group of ten volunteers made up of liver and kidney transplant recipients and their family members. Like many charitable organizations and groups that coalesce around specific chronic conditions, the Association was the product of personal suffering. The driving force behind it was Rosa Maria, the mother of two grown-up daughters with CKD, Carmen, twenty-five years of age, and Liza, eighteen. The girls were eight and one years old, respectively, when diagnosed with renal tubular acidosis, a condition which progressively worsened their kidney functioning. As Rosa Maria explained:

> They needed so much care, but we were told if they had a good nephrologist and a good nutritionist, they could have a good life. This was true. They have grown to be normal girls, able to participate in school and sports. They've had fun growing up. Both even had their transplants without needing dialysis. But like all problems that hurt like this one, all I wanted to know was "why *my* daughters?" Finally, you teach yourself to cope, to accept things as they are. Look, if this had never happened, I would never have started a project to help other people and now my daughter Carmen also works with us in the Association. She has grown up through this condition and has learned a positive life philosophy. You have to get the good out of the bad, right? . . . And that's the reason we started all this; those who are involved either have children that have been transplanted or are patients themselves. Many have lost children to this condition. When you have this problem, you are sensitive to the needs of people. We particularly want to help people cope and look after their health before their kidneys reach an end phase of functioning. Our plan is to grow, to have more resources and provide more support for people, not only medical care, but also psychological and emotional care, like promoting self-help therapy, maybe even other activities and classes, like dance classes or embroidery.

These longer term aspirations to support patients' wellbeing stood somewhat uneasily alongside the reactive firefighting the Association actually did in responding to the immediate needs of patients. What absorbed and constituted the main focus of its work was providing money, medications, biopsy needles, catheters, information, introductions to medical staff, clothes for those who had travelled to the city from neighboring states, and occasionally, when there was a surplus of time and resource, emotional and mental health support, although only on Saturday mornings when a volunteer psychologist was available to help. Approximately fifty kidney patients, at various stages of treatment, were dependent on the work of the Association at the time of interview, the majority trying to access a stable supply of medications, in particular, the immunosuppressant drug cyclosporine. Maintaining a ready supply of medications was not easy, so volunteer staff were continually negotiating with pharmacies and pharmaceutical companies, asking for samples, near to sell-by-date drugs, and donations.

It was not only uninsured patients who were dependent on this supply. Sometimes, insured patients from IMSS came to request medications, when faced with delays or shortages in the IMSS pharmacies. At the same time, patients from IMSS donated medications if they were given more than they needed, but these generally tended to be cheaper medications for hypertension or diabetes, rather than the more expensive cyclosporine. Speaking of immunosuppressant medication, Rosa Maria felt that the Association needed to invest in educating patients, suggesting that many lose their transplants because they failed to take immunosuppressants properly or did not maintain follow-up medical appointments. It is important, she explained, articulating a sentiment now worn out by its over-use, that families fully understand the gift they have received and know how to take care of it, to keep it as long as possible, reminding me that organ transplants do not last forever. However, at the same time, she explained that the challenges of living with CKD are not always addressed by ensuring that patients and their families are given the right information:

> Right now, we have a girl who has CKD and Tourette's. She is fifteen years old. Her parents cannot read or write and a number of the other family members already have CKD. We are trying to support this family so that they can get the tests done for an organ transplant. We are helping to coordinate the work they have to do, as well as help raise money for them. This little girl wants to live and we are going to support her. I feel we have adopted her. Already there have been so many problems. The family had started the protocols for transplantation four times now, but because the parents can't read or write, they struggle to keep their medical information with them. They often lose their test results, or don't bring in the correct paper-work for appointments, so now we are trying to accompany them to their appointments.

The greater part of Rosa Maria's and her colleagues' efforts was on supporting young people with the condition. It worried her that few of them knew why they had developed CKD. Earlier that day, she saw fourteen-year-old Sarai, who came into the office with her mother. Both were crying. Sarai's kidneys were in the end stages of functioning. She had recently been diagnosed and was required to have a series of tests but could not pay for them. Sarai was typical of the patients the

Association works with, referred to them by social workers or medical staff when hospitals ran out of their own options.

Developing the Association was not easy and required the building of dedicated networks of support and funding streams. To do this, connections had to be built with other charitable bodies who could act as advisors and teach them the work of being a charity, such as how to build a well-functioning organization, how to win allies, how to source the right suppliers, how to negotiate prices for medications and materials, how to write successful funding applications, how to campaign for the needs of their constituents, how to build a donor base, and so on. Alliances are all important for charitable associations and so the Association was a member of a city-wide network of charities who work for mutual benefit and share good practice. They had also initiated a new donor program which encouraged people to become *padrinos* (godparents) of the Association and donate a monthly sum.

In consolidating their work, they knew how important it was to have a good project, one which was credible, legitimate, and transparent. They also knew they had to be accountable and evidence their successes. This bureaucratization of giving embodies processes increasingly seen elsewhere, particularly in contexts where state forms of welfare have been eroded, giving way to more mixed forms of assistance put in place by the efforts of so-motivated individuals on a voluntary, not statutory basis. In the context of the increasing structural need for long-term, sustainable, and resource-intensive healthcare, individuals acting as individuals (even collectively) will only be able to help some, not all, and only in circumscribed ways, despite their best intentions and good work. Their efforts tend to work to sustain regimes of renal care on their terms, rather than on the terms of those who are dependent on them. In responding to problems with structural roots, problems created elsewhere and by others, and restricted to offering triage not restitution, these efforts tend to be conservative and preservative of a damaging status quo. This is an issue characteristic of charitable giving along the spectrum, from modest local endeavors to more elite forms (Erickson 2016; Hanson 2015). As Esping-Andersen (1990) notes, there is very little reason to believe that societies that cannot support provision to those in need collectively will be in a position to support it through the efforts of individuals. Quite the reverse: even the most energetic networks of individuals will quickly come up against the limits of their resources if they are operating in a social, political, and economic context where need has been generalized and made productive.

This is not to say that some individuals are not better placed to help than others. At the elite end of Mexico's spectrum of giving is the heavily promoted philanthropic work of the Carlos Slim Foundation. Regularly vying with people like Jeff Bezos, Bill Gates, Warren Buffet, and Mark Zuckerberg for the title of the world's richest person, Carlos Slim is a Mexican entrepreneur who amassed a $74 billion fortune, in large part due to his takeover of the previously state-owned phone company Telmex, following its privatization in 1990. Alongside building his significant business holdings, he also established a number of charitable initiatives in support of kidney disease and organ transplantation. As with Rosa Maria, his foundation also emerged out of personal tragedy. His wife Soumaya had died of kidney disease soon after a kidney transplant in 1999. His son Patrick was diagnosed with the condition in 2008, later transplanted with a kidney donated by another son. Through the Carlos Slim Foundation, the Carlos Slim Health Institute and a further initiative, *Héroes por la Vida* (Heroes for Life), Slim has worked with state governments, National Institutes of Health, hospital and civil society organizations to support 9,040 transplants, spending an estimated $20 million on the condition since 2001. Nevertheless, whether operating in the modest terms of the Association or those of an elite donor like Slim, charity does not make up for the limitations that renal care has revealed in Mexico, nor does it address its causes. Staying clear of the politics of health and poverty, the conditions out of which an impoverished healthcare infrastructure takes shape, and although they are proximate to social problems, charitable organizations are rarely instruments for social advocacy and political change. In the case of the Slim Foundation, they explicitly prefer to operate well outside these frames. One consequence of this is that they start to embody the very logics of scarcity that serve to patch people up and turn them into sites for the extraction of surplus value for others. These are the logics that keep transplant medicine alive and stop it (rather than the organs it depends on) from being rejected from the social body.

In her provocative paper, "The Impulse of Philanthropy," Erica Bornstein (2009) notes how the shifting registers of giving have intersected with contemporary notions of social responsibility, producing new forms of philanthropy and biosociality, in conjunction with new forms of neoliberal self-governance that valorize choice, autonomy, and empowerment (Miller and Rose 2008; Trnka and Trundle 2014). Accommodating the "impulse" to give within new systems of rational accountability and social responsibility reinforces the very same social inequalities that charitable giving hopes to mitigate (Bornstein 2009). This is because forms of organized charitable giving are predicated on class values that insist on worthiness, compliance, and appropriate expressions of gratitude on behalf of the recipient. Moreover, they do not confer any rights to recipients who, in turn, can make no claim on their donors. The lack of parity and the asymmetries between giver and receiver that charitable giving rests on resonates with the social obligations and expectations bound up with receiving an organ transplant more broadly. As I and others have written, the idea of organs as gifts, no less than what access to the care transplant medicine requires, exerts a moral pressure on the receiver to be grateful, to be well and healthy when they are not, to be independent, to be champions for organ donation campaigns, ultimately to be a good patient. The pressures and responsibilities bound to the so-called "gift of life" can, at times, be unbearable (Crowley-Matoka 2005; Kierans 2005, 2011; Sharp 2006;

Shimazono 2008). As Mary Douglas writing on Mauss makes clear, one does not get something for nothing (Douglas 1990), and the price demanded may exceed the benefits accrued.

The reproduction of inequality through charity is more stridently expressed by John Hanson in "An Anthropology of Giving" (2015), particularly with regard to forms of elite giving. Hanson describes elite giving as a system of domination, one in which charity is a rationalization of privilege. Ultimately, he suggests, quoting Sahlins, an elite charity's command of social capital will always "unbalance the flow of wealth in favor of the apparatus," a psychic magic or *Hau* in Mauss's terms, which impels the gift to return to its donor (Hanson 2015, 511). Charitable or philanthropic giving aligns people of similar social class backgrounds, enabling those that serve or manage such organizations to work effectively with healthcare professionals, politicians, and business elites, drawing together the motivations, values and assumptions of status hierarchies with regard to the needs of the disenfranchised. This is not to suggest that no good is performed, only that when various forms of giving emerge in the context of state denials of responsibility, we need to be cognizant of their multiple overlapping forms; their benefits but also their limits and through them their negative consequences.

Civil society organizations are a relatively recent phenomenon in Mexico (Escobar and Alvarez 1992; Hayden 2007a; Verduzco 2003). They emerged in the mid-1980s as part of a neoliberalizing state, one which loosened the grip of the Catholic Church and the corporatist state. Their relative late-comer status has been thought to explain why Mexico has a "charity-gap." A country with the lowest taxes and one of the highest income inequality rates among OECD (Organisation for Economic Co-operation and Development) nations, the percentage of Mexico's GDP dedicated to charity was 0.04 percent in 2003, increasing to 0.18 percent in 2009, a figure that falls substantially below that of Mexico's Latin American neighbors. Nonetheless, the spread of civil society and mutual assistance organizations has generated a new space for social action, a space that Gustavo Verduzco (2003) calls *lo público*, one which, in turn, has facilitated the financialization of new markets in healthcare. In this hybridized political economy of health and welfare, the urge to give and to profit are socially entangled (Trnka and Trundle 2014), yielding new forms of surplus from the social ruins of welfare.

THE FINANCIALIZATION OF GIVING: THE INTERPENETRATION OF GIFTS AND COMMODITIES

The life of a CKD patient is forever characterized by dependence on a varied array of medications; even after transplant surgery, this dependence never stops.[2] In fact, it becomes all the more critical and expensive. The *farmacia*—pharmacies and pharmacological enterprises where medications are supplied—are significant, though ambivalent, transactional and translational relays in the transplant supply

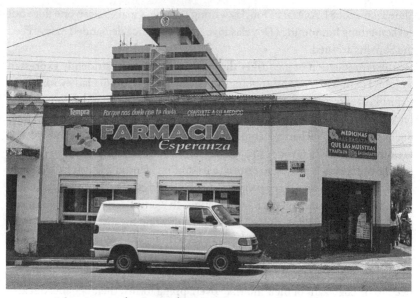

FIGURE 7. Advertisement (to the right) for "Medicinas Mas Baratas Que Las Muestras."

chain. They mediate and articulate the changing statuses kidney patients inhabit and provide another lens onto the multiple modes of exchange that coalesce around this condition.

The streets all around the perimeter of the public hospital are full of pharmacies—some well-established family businesses, some city-wide chains, and some simply new entrepreneurial ventures, all jostling in competition to serve an ever-expanding customer base. Their respective strategies for under-cutting each other, as figure 7 illustrates—"Medicinas Mas Baratas Que Las Muestras"—some of the medications they offer are even cheaper than the "free" samples handed out by pharmaceutical reps. Farmacia CARE was a family-owned pharmacy, nestled within this burgeoning medications market, positioned on a street corner directly opposite the public hospital. The premises were rented from a local church in the 1960s by Luis, the father of the current owner Daniel, and later bought outright by the family. Daniel was one of four brothers, all pharmacists, all running their own businesses. As a family, they have a long-standing relationship with the public hospital, its staff, and its patients, who they see on a daily basis. Their grandmother died in the hospital's leprosarium, leaving her daughter, their mother, orphaned, to be brought up under the care of the hospital's chaplain. The family see themselves and their business as part of the hospital's history. The hospital, in turn, constitutes approximately 55–60 percent of the pharmacy's sales, mostly through "walk-ins" (individuals coming in with their prescriptions), with the rest made up from orders from private hospitals and other pharma-related enterprises.

The pharmacy tries to keep costs down for poorer patients and charities. Reductions are provided by ensuring that supplies are bought direct through established contacts with manufacturers. However, these efforts are increasingly constrained by the expansion of the pharmaceutical sector and the imperative to maintain a competitive advantage. New pharmaceutical companies like PiSA and large pharmacy chains specializing in generics such as Farmacias Similares (Hayden 2007a) are now big players within the medicines market, against whom family businesses like CARE struggle to retain their market share.[3] Even more problematic is the extensive black market in medications, whose operations have engulfed the nearby Barrio de El Santuario, only three blocks away from the public hospital. Daniel explains:

> This underground selling of medications has, at least, a thirty-year history, but up until about ten years ago, it was a relatively small problem. Now it has completely taken over the streets with more and more new suppliers setting up businesses. Every year they get closer and closer to the hospital. And despite some efforts by the police to stop them, they continue to grow. This is really a big challenge for smaller family businesses like us. Just last week, I saw a person illegally selling on the street corner in front of the Faculty of Medicine. They are encroaching all the time and they are not afraid. COFEPRIS [Comisión Federal para la Protección contra Riesgos Sanitarios, the Federal Commission for the Protection against Sanitary Risks, which regulates medications] are not doing much. Either they don't have the capacity, are lazy or are colluding. And yet, while we are penalized if we don't conduct our business properly, like not maintaining the right refrigeration standards, this black market can continue right under our noses. There are zero rules. I have written to the Ministry for Health, but nothing happens. There is nothing I can do. I hold no authority. All of this illegal buying and selling is a consequence of a country like Mexico, one with no rules for those with the most connections.

Daniel regularly sees stacks of boxes from some of his more trusted suppliers piled high on the pavements by street sellers, suggesting to him a very well-organized market is at play that entwines legal and quasi-legal elements. From the perspective of the patient-buyer, street selling is both flexible and organized, easy to observe and navigate just by taking a short walk around the area. Labelling this activity "underground" is misleading. Business is conducted in full view and at all hours of the day only a short distance from the hospital, on one side of the city's main thoroughfares. At first glance, it looks like a collection of small "pop-up" shops—somewhere between thirty and forty in total—which have colonized a series of interconnected residential streets, nested into private houses or bolted onto existing small businesses. The entire operation is supplemented by individual dealers who cover a wide radius outward from the hospital and who facilitate sales remotely. Outside their provisional premises, small groups sit on plastic chairs talking to customers or placing orders on their mobile phones. All social classes are represented on either side of these transactions. Even at a glance, the passer-by will note its relatively sophisticated logistical operation. Sellers call out continually, asking all passers-by what they are looking for.

On one occasion, while walking around this neighborhood, Cesar and I asked for erythropoietin (EPO), a synthetic hormone that promotes the formation of red blood cells, often prescribed for CKD patients with anemia. We were immediately given a reduced price of 500 pesos (40 U.S. dollars). Despite being illegal, street selling was well-organized, well-known, and habitually used. In many ways, it had the feel of a *tianguis* (a street market for food and household goods), nothing particularly out of the ordinary, and the authorities too acted as if that were the case. During one of our visits, a police car drove past, slowed down, took a quick look down one of the streets, turned a corner, sped up, and was on its way again. We were told there were few raids on these premises, and when they did happen, businesses closed quickly and resumed as normal the following day. Even a more sustained period of policing designed to push sellers away from the immediate environs of the public hospital, which saw a police cordon sanitaire ringing the hospital in a five-block radius, did little more than relocate the market. Rumors quickly circulated that this was because deals had been made which were designed to secure the position of "legitimate" dealers every bit as dubious as the black-market dealerships, just less visibly so.

Daniel explained the success of street selling as capitalizing on an opportunity presented by poverty:

> People simply do not have money, which makes it easy for a black market to thrive—what choices do patients have? They have to buy medications where they can find them cheapest. I don't judge them. But we try to explain to them that they do this at their own risk and that they should never buy medications that they do not trust, no matter how cheap. But it doesn't make any difference. I think it is because we do not have a culture of protecting health . . . Health is way down the list.

Currently, Daniel's pharmacy is helping to support eighteen families with CKD, mostly by providing low cost medication and supplies, but also by being part of much wider networks of charitable support and advice. Trying to provide medication at an affordable cost for people is not, he explains, straightforward.

> So for example, we have to work with what the doctor prescribes—I cannot, by law, alter or change a prescription, but I do what I can to make it as cheap as possible and when I can't do this, I have an agreement with some of the civil

associations, where they will agree to support the costs of medications, or we direct the patient to DIF's development programs, or to Caritas. I also have long-term relationships with some of the laboratories—and so we are continually providing links and information, so that patients can find good options. We now know all the associations who support specific diseases, like cancer or CKD. And, we work closely with the social work department in the hospital who assess patients and put them in contact with different sources of help and support.

Lowering costs is inevitably done in consideration of accounting for business overheads and profit margins which, Daniel explains, they minimally keep at between 10 and 12 percent. However, profits on some items, like catheters, are sacrificed. These are bought in volume and used to negotiate business arrangements with clinical specialties such as nephrology in order to build good will and positive working relationships. After forty years in the business, Daniel says they are still looking for ways to improve, but he also states that they try to stick to principles that are based on respect for the needs of people, particularly the poor, and to accommodate them within their business model.

The rhetoric of poverty and social need, as a context for business, was one that emerged regularly in interviews and discussions with those working in medical supplies and pharmaceutical enterprises. The idea that publics without entitlement have become the foundation for a new pharmaceutical business model is one that has not gone unnoticed by other anthropologists working in Mexico. Cori Hayden (2007a) explicitly focused on this issue in her analysis of the well-known Mexican pharmaceutical chain Farmacias Similares, one of the more visible actors in the circulation of cheaper, copied pharmaceuticals in the country.[4] Farmacias Similares's efforts to harness and grow a national generic drugs industry have been described as a populist privatization, exemplified by the tag line, "Mexican Products to Help Those Who Have the Least." The growth of Farmacias Similares is attributed to its ability to undermine the hegemonic power of global pharmaceutical companies who were selling their expensive branded drugs to the Mexican market. As Hayden points out, the drugs produced and sold under the Similares name undercut their branded counterparts by being 75 percent cheaper. Their capacity to do so has to be seen in the context of the medication shortages and rising drugs costs that characterized healthcare in Mexico during the late 1990s and that acted as a spur to the Mexican government, health activists, and the private sector to drive forward the production of generic drugs. These moves were readily articulated as acting in the public interest and achieved by transforming a poor and unentitled public into a capitalist-friendly market alternative, assisting, in turn, the privatization of the provision of healthcare in Mexico (Hayden 2007a). Hayden states that "efforts to create new pharmaceutical markets are nothing if not projects of invoking and producing a certain notion of the 'the people' in a decidedly political and populist sense" (2007a, 484). They show, she asserts, the mutual constituting forces of public and private interests in new markets in healthcare.

In turning back to the growing population of uninsured CKD sufferers, the opportunities for capitalizing on public need remain significant. Although this constituency of uninsured poor patients have not been as explicitly invoked by the engulfing renal supplies and medications market—as is the case with Farmacias Similares—they have nonetheless been recognized as a significant consumer base, however mediated by a broad coalition of donor organizations and healthcare providers. Those who are poor, fragmented, disenfranchised, and dependent are easily harnessed to new infrastructures of giving, care, and support. Taking Hayden's point, this has provided fertile conditions for financialization and opportunities for capital through the transformation of heretofore non-market activities (i.e., the work of families, charities, civil society organizations, etc.) into sites of profit making. Put another way, the harms inflicted on Mexico's uninsured, set in train by welfare state failures, has generated a haphazardly articulated assemblage of gifts and commodities, which draws informal and charitable giving into the logics and plans of market actors. These new market forms have colonized the relationship between state and society, between private and public realms, making them permeable and, most significantly, rendering them transactional and thus exploitable.

These complex and entangled supply chains harnessed to ideas of public good and public health were best exemplified by Guillermo Hernandez, a regional manager for the Mexican pharmaceutical corporation PiSA. PiSA is a Mexican pharmaceutical company that has been producing renal-related medical products for over twenty-five years. The company started by producing peritoneal dialysis solutions and, soon after, products for hemodialysis and transplant medicine. More recently, it has moved into the arena of diabetes medicines in an attempt to build "synergy" into their operations and ultimately to develop a line of pre-dialysis products that would cover the entire patient trajectory. Since its inception, it has worked closely with healthcare professionals, organizing and financially supporting scientific and clinical talks, symposiums, and events.

In a similar vein to Hayden's account of Farmacias Similares, PiSA entered into the Mexican pharma market to challenge the hold transnational corporations had on Mexican product and supply chains. In this case, it was the globalized brand, Baxter, which had held the monopoly on dialysis supplies in Mexico until PiSA entered the market. Guillermo explained:

> When PiSA Laboratories entered the market, they were directly confronting Baxter. PiSA was a family owned company based in Jalisco, daring to challenge what was a powerful monopoly. It was a battle which lasted for many years, and one unknown to many people. Baxter was anti-competitive. Instead of challenging us with quality or clinical efficiency, the company used patient support groups to

speak against our products. They even supported them to demonstrate outside IMSS hospitals, saying "PiSA's products are killing us; they want to kill us; they want us to die." At that time, renal patients undergoing CAPD had to pick up their own dialysate boxes and bring them to their homes. A poor patient had to hire a number of taxis to take all the boxes they would need for a month, adding additional costs to their treatments. Baxter had developed a home delivery system in other countries, but it wasn't available in Mexico, because it came with a cost. It was only when PiSA entered the market that Baxter started their home deliveries.

The supply and distribution of home dialysis products became part of a strategy to gain a competitive advantage by both companies. This was supplemented by the provision of other supports, such as, temporary "cabins" for patients who had no space to perform dialysis at home, and home visits by dialysis nurses to oversee the various ways dialysis was implemented in the home.

Stepping up on innovation gave PiSA an advantage, forcing the company into new modes of production, quality procedures, and standards. PiSA expanded into the hemodialysis market after consolidating its peritoneal dialysis enterprise and, according to Guillermo, provided patients and healthcare professionals with more choice than ever before. Its business model relies on a network of close working relations that focuses not only on the end consumer, namely the hospital, clinic, or home dialysis user, but on all those who mediate and facilitate the distribution and supply of dialysis productions, such as charities, civil society associations, and support groups. Guillermo continues:

I work closely with many charities. We have supported almost forty of them, some registered charities, others unregistered, but all working for the benefit of patients. We support them with medicines and medical supplies, provide financial support to others, and have given talks to many of them. We have a special agreement of collaboration with one foundation, which includes price reductions . . . We encourage them to choose the options they think are the best for them. With another association, we have been able to position and direct our supplies of erythropoietin as well as other medicines. We also have a contract to provide outsourced hemodialysis treatments in conjunction with a charity who operates several hemodialysis clinics in different Mexican cities.

. . . We also work closely with Fundación Telmex [a Carlos Slim foundation], supplying products to their dialysis programs. Fundación Telmex has peritoneal dialysis, hemodialysis, and transplantation programs in a number of hospitals across the country. I would say that Fundación Telmex is the most important charity in Mexico, certainly the most active in supporting renal patients. And they support everything, transplantation, dialysis programs, surgeries, and so on. They are really socially committed to this cause . . .

... In working with charities, we have developed outreach strategies, because we do not only produce medicines and dialysis solutions, we also work to bring these products to patients. For instance, in our company's drugstores, Farmacia La Paz, we offer discounts to patients who are supported by charities. They only have to show proof of that support and demonstrate that the medicines are for them. Just as an example, erythropoietin has a market price of around 2,800 pesos [224 U.S. dollars], but we know it can be bought for 600 pesos [48 U.S. dollars] on the streets. So we have tried to provide support at this level to people particularly through the charities [in effect undercutting the street vendors].

Guillermo is fully aware of his company's role in the provision of public health, knowing that so many different kinds of healthcare institutions are now full of CKD patients but have limited resources to tackle this growing problem. He is also clear that this patient population requires more and more support from charities, in order to extend the reach of clinics and hospitals to patients in need. He is acutely aware that no one can transplant their way out of this problem and that kidney patients will remain kidney patients regardless. This also means that rigorous regimes of pharmaceutical care will continue.

With the public's health in mind, the challenge for Guillermo is to continue to increase the market share in every area where PiSA has a stake. The company would like to multiply the number of hemodialysis clinics in Mexico extending them from six to fifty clinics in the next two years. It currently produces just one type of peritoneal dialysis solution, one which is glucose based, but it would like to introduce more specialized solutions to the market, ones modified in calcium and magnesium, with added amino acids and that are glucose free. With regard to transplant medicine, its big challenge is to devise and offer a comprehensive therapy with the full range of immunosuppressants and, similarly, for peritoneal dialysis and hemodialysis patients, it wants to extend the business into the production of nutrients, such as L-carnitine, iron, vitamin C, and vitamin B. The company's ambitions are far from modest, but fully in line with the range of therapies and medicines renal patients require. In this, Guillermo explains, it wants to be the single supplier, an ambition articulated as much through the language of markets and profits as of social responsibility and quality of care.

The compromised, multiply-hybridized character of the actually existing forms of exchange that transplantable and failing organs incorporate function between patients, kin, and community; charitable bodies (of all sizes); street vendors, pharmaceutical, and medical suppliers (national and transnational); hospitals, clinics, and healthcare professionals (public and private); and the wider governmental arrangements in which they are anchored (from finance ministries, through welfare systems to public and commercial law-making). Being so hybridized, they create difficulties in working with attenuated use-value and exchange-value distinctions associated with structuralist or classical political economy perspectives (for further discussion see Foster 2011; Tsing 2009, 2013). These forms of exchange teach us that value(s) cannot be automatically attributed to organs as things to be exchanged—in non-market or market terms—as gifts or commodities. They point us instead to how particular sited processes of exchange, and the social relations that underpin them, create the conditions for value production, a form of production parasitic on the ordinary labor and bios of others (Jones and Mair 2016). Further, the exploitation of such labor and the transformation of harm and suffering into opportunities for capital are neither static nor uniform (Taussig 1980; Wolf 1982). What these multiple forms of exchange also teach us is that regimes of renal care overspill and spread out into the wider culture, society, political system, and economy, but also that cultural, social, political, and economic practices have been reconfigured so that people can respond to, invest in, or capitalize on that overspill.

Anna Tsing (2013) takes up these multiple forms of exchange by focusing on the heterarchical relations of production and exchange that underpin the supply and transformation of a very different object of exchange—the Matsutake mushroom. Studying its supply chains, Tsing questions the taken-for-granted logics at play when commodities are understood to define the value system under capitalism "with little consideration of the processes of transformation that they undergo" (2013, 22). She demonstrates the importance of understanding how the production and exchange of things internally relate to value production. This helps her to examine the economic heterogeneities that underpin capital, rather than treat them as processes which are already pre-formed and determining in character. Organs similarly rely on intricate and entangled forms of gift and commodity exchange in order to pull into orbit around them a complex and locally adapted system of exchange logics, one which produces capital for others. These processes of transformation, to borrow from Appadurai, might be described as "tournaments of value," "complex periodic events that are removed in some culturally well-defined way from the routines of economic life" but are nevertheless central to it (Appadurai 1986, 21).

Although the value produced by the appropriated labor of poor Mexican families might well be removed from the routines of economic life, it paradoxically suggests a "pure," fully disembedded and thus abstract form of capitalism, because those who labor to produce organs-for-transplant do so in the absence of any capacity (or requirement) to reproduce their own efforts. In this case, the production of value is vampiric. It works in the space where labor is directed to maintaining life; by staving off its end, it extracts without restoration. The profound struggle by living-related organ donors and recipients to stay alive is, therefore, the very basis for the production of profit, and the primary activity that animates transplant medicine too. All that flows from this only serves to diminish the capacity of those affected—not just the patient and their extended families but wider society—to ensure that health is protected and everyday lives reproduced. In the absence of adequate social protections, and where an emphasis on rights and entitlements is little more than rhetorical, those with the least resources to expend on their health often do so to the point of utter depletion. Arendt argues that "the human capacity for life in the world always implies an ability to transcend and to be alienated from the processes of life itself, while vitality and liveliness can be conserved only to the extent that men are willing to take the burden, the toil and trouble of life, upon themselves" (1998 [1958], 120). The problem with contemporary transplant medicine in Mexico is that while the poor are obliged to take on that burden, and others profit from them doing so, they are consumed by it. In this way, to adapt Habermas (1984), the colonization of the life-world of poor Mexicans by organ transplantation wreaks profound damage on them for the benefit of others.

With poverty a key player in Mexican medical markets, with minimally half of the population without welfare entitlements and a steady proportion of those with entitlements suffering under a system already at breaking point, the surplus activity thus produced and transformed into more rationalized processes by the work of charities and philanthropic associations generates a new resource to be harnessed in the incongruous entanglements between public health and capital. This surplus activity reworks the gift/commodity distinction, producing value through unplanned contingency, reconfiguring poverty and inequality into a *tercer via* (third way) healthcare market. Here profit and poverty sit comfortably together: one allows for and underpins the other.

When considering regimes of renal care, what we are *not* seeing is the extensions of new medical technologies under capitalism. This is not primarily about systems of exploitation founded on the profit motive or the superior role of the market. Nor indeed should we treat the growth of renal care as a function of the state and its systems of governmentality or legibility. What we are seeing are the many ways in which state, market, and society mutually implicate and shape one another. The modes of exchange underpinning organ transplantation cannot be pre-figured. There is no given or prescribed platform in Mexico from which transplant medicine can be said to work or which could provide a vantage point for an authoritative or organizational overview of the processes of organ exchange—the donation and receipt of organs. The very messiness of transplant medicine stabilizes it; the only vantage points available are those accessed by entering into that mess. When we abandon the external for the internal viewpoint, we learn about organ transplantation as an outcome of the very exchanges that enable it to form and grow. These are difficult to see all at once—and even with detailed ethnographic work, certain elements will continue to recede from view. However, every now and then, it is possible to expose multiple layers, even all at once. The enterprises and social actors who pull various forms of exchange together, for example, the pharmacies and pharmaceutical companies; doctors, nurses, and social workers; scientists and lab technicians; politicians; charitable bodies, and philanthropic foundations; family, friends, and neighbors, among others, show us something about the character of exchange at many levels, from the ordinary to the elite. It would be inaccurate to see these, however, solely in economic terms; their political currencies too are important. Engaging with the internal politics of transplant medicine provides another important internal vantage point from which to get its measure. This is a point the next chapter will attest.

6 · TRANSPLANT SCANDALS, THE STATE, AND THE "MULTIPLE PROBLEMATICS" OF ACCOUNTABILITY

In 2008, Hospital Civil was embroiled in a widely publicized, but somewhat ambiguous, corruption scandal centered on organ exchange. The hospital had attracted one of the country's top surgeons, Dr. Luis Carlos Rodríguez Sancho, medically trained at the prestigious Mayo Clinic in the United States. He had been invited to work in the city about ten years before by a prominent PRD politician, someone who held a number of high profile directorships within the city's medical and educational institutions and who was keen to support and enhance the development of the city's expanding organ transplant programs.[1] Upon his arrival in Guadalajara, the surgeon appeared, almost single handedly, to accelerate the pace and rate of organ transplantation, establishing a deceased organ donation and transplant program to enhance the transplantation of livers and kidneys. The blurring of the lines that link supply and demand, donation and use of organs, foreshadowed the later controversies that would arise around his medical practices.

In 2008, the surgeon was suspended from his post. He was reputed to have accepted substantial payments for transplanting private patients who had not been on recognized transplant waiting lists, amid rumors of organ trafficking and corruption. The events that followed culminated in a rupture between the living-organ and cadaveric transplant programs and their respective teams, while serving to make visible a series of political interconnections between university, medical, and city leaders and their mutually informing practices of governance.

Although these events occurred three years before my ethnographic fieldwork commenced, their effects were still keenly felt during it. The scandal, with its allegations of corrupt practice, provided a window, which many would have wished to remain shut, onto the socio-political arrangements that underpinned the

governance and organizational development of transplant medicine. It showed
the tangled ways in which transplant medicine was made to work both inside and
outside of the functional space of the clinic. From an ethnographic point of view,
the events that took place in 2008 significantly shaped what those working in the
hospital were prepared to say when interviewed. Nevertheless, through the col-
lusions, alliances, and disputes that followed, it was possible to see the wider
operations of organ transplantation, as itself a collaborative ethnographic project,
where different social actors create the limits and possibilities of medical technologies and establish the norms through which they work based on descriptions,
analyses, and achieved understandings of the situations they were in.

In this chapter, I reconstruct the collaborative ethnographic work of others
(doctors, institutional directors, politicians, journalists, for example) as an instance
of what Holmes and Marcus (2008) describe as ethnographies of alignment.
The idea of alignment sensitizes us to the fact that our ethnographic subjects
are engaged in intellectual labors and ways of sense-making often indistinguish-
able from those employed by anthropologists. They are intellectually navigating
the same terrain that we are. In examining the events of 2008, first, I consider what
different accounts of this scandal can teach us about the socio-political context
within which transplant medicine is made to work. I am particularly interested in
how a politics is revealed when things go wrong; when we are invariably taken
beyond the medical into the domains of state-work (legal, disciplinary, and regulatory). As a consequence, I ask, in examining these accounts, how the state is
invoked in this context. Second, I consider the ways in which medical scandals as
"extraordinary" events can cast light on what is considered to be their opposite:
the ordinary, mundane, or normative practices of technological medicine. In so
doing, I suggest that this particular scandal served to render locally organized,
everyday forms of transplant medicine ordinary, even when those ordinary ways
of working can be seen, when approached slightly differently, as anything but. In
outlining my approach, my point is not to report on a scandal for its own sake, to
establish what did or did not definitively occur, or to arbitrate between different
versions of events. I aim rather to examine how the event was mobilized, by whom,
and for what purposes, and through that to reflect on the lessons such incidents
can teach us about the political character of organ transplantation and its interfacing and intersecting interests.

ON SCANDALS AND CORRUPT ACTIVITIES

The organ scandal has, in recent years, become a common trope, one used to structure accounts of transplant medicine across anthropological literatures. It serves
to organize understandings of biotechnical modes of exchange: the various ways
in which organs and tissues come to be procured, retained, and allocated, and
upon which the transplant project itself, in many respects, hinges. The forms of

exchange that underpin the transfer of organs have been claimed, time and again, to be vulnerable to abuses of trust, power, and the misappropriation of public resources, and so have been readily connected to issues of malpractice and the unequal production of health and harm across global settings (Ikels 2013; Nguyen and Peschard 2003; Scheper-Hughes 2000). Nancy Scheper-Hughes's work on the subject is without question the best known, both inside and outside the field of anthropology. With extensive publications dedicated to the organ trade alone, her work is seen by some as path breaking, a triumph of the anthropological endeavor, but by others, as remarked by Roy D'Andrade (1995, 408), as a form of "estheticized journalism and moralistic pamphleteering." While I do not propose to revisit her varied and variable contributions, Scheper-Hughes's research suggests that there are dangers in sensationalizing problems of organ procurement. As Marilyn Strathern (2009) notes, dramatizing subjects that seem made for drama can detract from rather than add to our understanding. Such, however, is the ubiquity of scandals in various accounts of transplant medicine that many people I spoke to about my research invariably assumed this is what drew me to both the subject and the field site. Although this was not the case, scandals and the corrupt activities that sustain them are present and important. In the context of this study, they are critical heuristics in the analysis of institutional practice and, for that reason, cannot be ignored. Here anthropology provides fewer resources than one might imagine, particularly for the analysis of the practices of corruption and malpractice that scandals so often draw attention to (Torsello 2010). With the notable exception of James Scott's (1972) work on political corruption, anthropologists have contributed little to debates on the subject (Haller and Shore 2005).

This is, perhaps, not surprising. Corruption is not an easy subject for anthropologists to engage with, not least because practices of corruption do not readily lend themselves to ethnographic modes of engagement—with an emphasis on "being there"—while raising significant safeguarding concerns for both the fieldworker and informants. Anthropologists have also been wary of the ways in which generalized accounts of corruption, particularly across the wider Anglophone social sciences, can fall foul of asymmetric analyses, with corrupt practice treated as synonymous with weak and unstable states, too easily linked to a non-Western "other" (Haller and Shore 2005). Mexico is particularly vulnerable to this form of othering. It is a country whose institutional processes have been historically naturalized as corrupt and positioned in stark comparison to more "legitimate" Anglo-European modes of operating (Whyte 2015; Haller and Shore 2005).

The tendency to view corruption in terms of simplifying moral binaries, for example, ordinary/extraordinary, legitimate/illegitimate, and global north/global south, suggests there is a need to maintain symmetry in ethnographic interpretation by attending to the social practices within which those binaries become descriptive as well as to the social practices that they describe (Bloor 1991). According to Haller and Shore (2005), we should not see corruption under its restrictive, provincial, and puritan guises, but as something subtle, layered, and complex. We need to grasp its politics and poetics, to recognize that what stands as corrupt in one setting may not carry over to another. Take, for example, practices of gift-giving, reciprocity, forms of patronage, clientelism, trust, and loyalty (Auyero 2000; Herzfeld 1992; Mauss 1990 [1950]; Sahlins 1963; Strathern 1974). On one reading, these ubiquitous forms of social exchange might be regarded as petty forms of corruption. On another, they can be fundamental to fortifying ambivalent relationships, galvanizing political allies, and ensuring social cohesion. They form part of the complex ways in which individuals and groups connect to the state and its administrative worksites as well as to each other (Gupta 2012). Rather than assuming corruption to be discrete and determinate, it may be more useful to think about what it "produces"—how it makes visible the social relations of institutional practice; how it generates various kinds of social actor (responsible or irresponsible), a rule of law, citizenship, and rights, and how, in so doing, it serves to demarcate the legitimate from the illegitimate, the ordinary from the extraordinary.

Studies of corruption provide an important lens on the constitution of social norms and institutional logics, by attending to their violations. In other words, the disruptive and controversial character of corruption makes available the constitutive elements of social institutions and the social relations that underpin them. As Gupta (1995) suggests, various forms of illicit activity require an institutional ground of social hierarchy and collective expectation against which they register—in other words, one that is ordinary and routine. If this is so, how might we identify and examine the ground that links ordinary and extraordinary practice as mutually constitutive? How does one provide an avenue for understanding the other? The transplant scandal affords us one way to tease this out. It teaches us something valuable about transplant medicine and the manner in which it is embedded in the institutional and organizational life of a hospital; the expectations for how it should function; what it should achieve, how it is to respond to the scarce resources it depends on; the uses and misuses of power and where; and whom people look to when things go wrong. As these concerns are brought to the surface, we see the complex interplay between medicine and the state, with the expansion of medical technologies as a particular type of political practice.

The morphology of the transplant scandal in Guadalajara unfolded as a chronologically shaped presentation of events, reported serially across city and state news media. This involved dailies like *Informador, Mural,* and *La Jornada*; weekly news magazines: *Proceso* and *Crítica*; and the television news programs of Televisa Guadalajara, TV Azteca's Hechos Jalisco and MegaNoticias. It was not, therefore, drawn from first-hand observations or from interviews with key protagonists, though it has been enhanced with reflections from my informants—both patients and doctors. In the context of fieldwork, the event was only discussed and recoverable in retrospect, so there was little direct access. Focusing instead on media reports of various kinds brings forth a different kind of analytical affordance. In attempting to understand how scandals serve to publicly link together systems of medical practice, power, and governance, reporting in the media, newspapers in particular, represents a valuable way to consider how these connections are publicly fashioned and the pieces fitted together.

THE TRANSPLANT SCANDAL

On 19 February 2008, Armida Mestas received a liver transplant in Hospital Civil. Prior to this, she had been receiving care for end stage liver disease at an ISSSTE specialty hospital in the city of Tepic, Nayarit, but one without liver transplant specialists. While there, one of her doctors recommended she contact the surgeon Luis Carlos Rodríguez Sancho, who was reputed to have revolutionized the transplant program at Hospital Civil. Armida's case was taken on by Dr. Rodríguez Sancho and arranged privately at a cost of 800,000 pesos (71,400 U.S. dollars). Her family were asked to make a down payment of 400,000 pesos (35,400 U.S. dollars) and sign off four promissory notes for 100,000 pesos (8,900 U.S. dollars) to be paid in monthly installments after the transplant had taken place. Her family re-mortgaged their house to do this. The money was then deposited in a personal bank account, later found out to be that of Dr. Rodríguez Sancho's father.

On 18 April, two months later, Armida Mestas died. Her family went to CETOT (the Jalisco State Council for Organ and Tissue Transplantation) to report what had happened. They claimed she had died as a result of medical negligence and had been abandoned by her doctors after experiencing post-transplant complications. As a result, they stopped paying the monthly installments.

Armida's case was not isolated. She was one of a number of patients who had been transplanted through the same set of financial arrangements and who were also in the process of lodging complaints with CETOT. On 10 March, one month prior to Armida's death, at the Annual Meeting of the Regional Organ Donation and Transplants Councils, the then director of CENATRA declared rumors of "misconduct" that implicated Rodríguez Sancho.[2] He was reported to be charging as much as one million pesos for a transplant without consulting the appropriate transplant committees, and to be working in collaboration with a hospital in a nearby state, which was rumored to be supplying him with livers. On 11 April 2008, the transplant program at Hospital Civil was officially suspended by CETOT.

On 4 July, *Mural,* one of the city's newspapers, broke the story with the headline, "Lucran con órganos en el Hospital Civil" (Profiting with organs at Hospital Civil); this was quickly followed on 6 July by an article in *Mural* which reported that the transplant program at the hospital had been suspended. On 10 July, an article in *Informador* was published under a more provocative title, "Arraigan Luis Carlos Rodríquez Sancho por presunto tráfico de orgános," suggesting that

Rodríquez Sancho had been placed under house arrest due to alleged organ traf-ficking. These were to be the first of thirty articles published by *Informador* on this issue, alongside in-depth coverage by the magazine *Proceso*, which also presented events at the hospital as a trafficking scandal. The issue received sustained cover-age across the city's various media for the next six months.

On 10 July, Rodríguez Sancho was placed under house arrest at the request of the state comptroller, Contraloria del Estado de Jalisco (the Office of the State Comptroller and General Auditor).[3] The arrest was in relation to organ traffick-ing allegations and the charging of private patients in a public hospital of between 800,000 and one million pesos for privileged access to livers and kidneys. A notice-able feature of the media's reporting would be the slippery, hard-to-define char-acter of the purported "wrongdoing." This was variously described by different reporters as *tráfico de órganos, delitos de responsabilidad médica; irregularidades administrativas; los delitos de peculado, desvío de recursos, responsabilidad médica,* or *el escándalo*—in other words, respectively, possible or alleged organ traffick-ing, crimes of medical liability, administrative irregularities, embezzlement, diver-sion of resources, malpractice, or, simply, a scandal. That a scandal had emerged was not in doubt. However, its precise shape, content, and causes were much less easily discerned.

The events in question would have far-reaching repercussions for the organ-ization, administration, and reputation of the institution's living-related and deceased transplant programs, which at the time of my research were operating as two separate entities, supported by two different but occasionally overlapping nephrology and transplant teams. As a consequence, the "facts of the matter" were communicated by those working in the hospital either obliquely or not at all. What was clear was that the issue itself would set conditions and boundaries to field-work: how it would be organized, what it was possible to learn, and from whom. The details of the case were widely and publicly known. Nevertheless, few of the medical staff were prepared to talk or to be seen talking about it, as loyalties as well as careers and career prospects were sensitive to the social relations of the medical community and its wider systems of governance and power that had been entangled in this particular controversy.

The investigations that ensued were also multiple and overlapping and involved a range of judicial, regulatory, and public institutions. Who came to have juris-diction over which aspects of alleged wrongdoing is revealing in its own right. The formal basis of investigations into the scandal were four complaints, all filed by relatives of transplant patients, made to the Contraloria del Estado de Jalisco, which launched an official investigation. The Contraloria is the institution responsible for disciplining public servants and the body responsible for issuing sanctions.

Accompanying this central investigation was an array of official and quasi-legal inquiries and processes. They included an investigation by the Procuraduría

General de Justicia de Jalisco (the police) who were looking into the explicit claim of organ trafficking. It was the police who placed the surgeon under house arrest as a potential flight risk. They also included an investigation by the Comisión Estatal de Derechos Humanos de Jalisco (the Jalisco State Human Rights Commission), which was approached independently by concerned patients and their families and by Rodríguez Sancho's lawyers, all claiming—albeit for different reasons—that their human rights had been violated. Conciencia Cívica Jalisciense (CCJ) also had a role to play. The CCJ was a local social justice NGO, run by a well-known former PRI politician, Cosío Gaona. He financially supported some of the patients in their legal action and made that support public. And finally, the Comisión Federal para la Protección contra Riesgos Sanitarios (COFEPRIS), the federal body for regulating against health risks, conducted an audit of the activities that took place at the hospital.

The various investigations and appeals for support were the subject of intense documentation, scrutiny, and reporting over the summer of 2008. As a body of public information, it did more than simply document the vagaries and developments of a public interest story; it also pulled into view an entire network of social actors and the political cleavages that defined their relationships. It is the particular character and consequences of these relationships on which I focus here. They help to make clear the social ground upon which local elaborations of organ transplantation rest and around which its cultural specificities take form.

THE INTERPLAY OF GOVERNMENTAL ACTORS

The implications of the scandal were not confined to the practices of one institution. Rather, it spread across the inter-institutional arrangements and politics that underpinned relations between the University of Guadalajara and the hospital. Both institutions shared a medical curriculum and their structures of governance incorporated many of the same local political leaders, individuals who had at various times assumed different positions across the city's political, educational, medical, and cultural institutions. This meant that the scandal implicated some of the city's most influential power brokers. In fact, the scandal emerged as a result of a well-publicized rift between the university's then rector, Carlos Briseño Torres, and Raul Padilla López, former rector general of the University of Guadalajara (1989–1995), someone who was regarded as the unofficial but de facto leader of the university, holding substantive power over Briseño Torres's office. A close ally of Padilla López's—Dr. Raul Vargas López—a prominent PRD politician and former director of Hospitales Civiles Trust (1997–2001), was responsible for Rodríguez Sancho's appointment in 1998. Briseño was said to have seized upon complaints and rumors about malpractice at the hospital in order to confront Padilla López and his associates and to wrest back control over affairs at the university.

Commentators suggested Briseño Torres wanted to create a firewall between the everyday institutional norms and working practices of the university and the hospital. In an *Informador* article of 10 July, titled "UdeG aguarda investigaciones en Hospital Civil" (the university awaits investigations at the hospital), the university rector asserted that the public hospital represented an *organismo público descentralizado* (a decentralized public institution), and that, despite shared teaching between the institutions, the university was not compromised by this event. Briseño Torres was particularly vociferous in his denouncements of the emerging scandal, calling for la Procuraduría del Estado to continue with its investigations *caiga quien caiga* (no matter who falls). This public break on the scandal between known political rivals was duly noted by the media, and provided rich material for speculation on the motives that drove it. In good analytic fashion, commentators focused not just on what the rivals were saying, but what they were attempting to do by saying it. Briseño Torres had provided a way in.

What followed were various and competing attempts to implicate the hospital and, in the process, Raul Padilla, through assertions that the surgeon acted with the full knowledge and support of hospital management and city authorities or, alternatively, assertions that the surgeon had acted alone and in his own personal interest. What was clear was that in the years leading up to the scandal, the hospital had benefitted from the dramatic rise in transplant surgeries. Thus, as news of the scandal broke across the city, it became more apparent that the heroic efforts to increase access to organs-for-transplant might be contingent on less than legitimate practices. Indeed, in the aftermath, the hospital's impressive transplant statistics started to fall, indexed by a decrease in both organs donated and organs transplanted. The whole affair inevitably raised concerns about the longer-term impact on the public's willingness to donate organs, as well as damage to the reputation of the hospital.

What made the scandal and its effects on the hospital particularly confusing was the lack of clarity over what had actually taken place: medical malpractice; embezzlement; organ trafficking; profiteering; something else? The ambiguities at the heart of the matter, so open to varying and competing interpretations, fueled extraordinary levels of speculation and recrimination, turning a political wheel into full spin and bringing a substantial cast of political, medical, and civic stakeholders into play.

Stances on the matter did not neatly divide into two camps. In some cases, the scandal provoked cautious and circumspect responses, in others, clear and unequivocal denunciations. Others still focused on what was at stake for the long term. A retired physician who had worked with CETOT—one of the few to share an opinion with me on the matter—talked about the need to protect the work and reputation of the public hospital. For him, there was the potential loss of a brilliant and talented surgeon, the reputational damage for an institution that had served the state's poor and disenfranchised for centuries, and the inevitable setback for an up-and-coming transplant program for which there was no short-age of local need, and which was nationally acclaimed.

Speaking for others with a stake in local healthcare, he suggested it was impor-tant that whatever irregularities were at play, those involved acted outside of the norm. Conventional hospital working procedures had not been followed, and that was the problem. Moreover, he suggested, the scandal or alleged wrongdoing and the institution within which it was said to have taken place were for him not one and the same thing. With that, he reflected on Briseño Torres's role in publiciz-ing the whole affair. From his perspective, Briseño Torres had produced the scan-dal. It was he who named it, he who brought it to public attention. This physician felt the entire situation could have been dealt with more diplomatically, without giving rise to a media circus that impacted negatively on the university, the hos-pital and its staff, and on affiliated organizations like CETOT. There was clearly much at stake for all in question, and the lack of clarity around the surgeon's actions did not make it easy to quell speculation, no matter how far from the hospital the problems surfaced. As the physician implied, given the interpretive room that had been generated, whatever had actually happened at the hospital, could be taken up and publicly pursued for all manner of political ends and means.

ESTABLISHING WHO KNEW WHAT

The very public nature of the scandal ensured that those with a stake in preserv-ing the status and reputation of the hospital and transplant program quickly entered the frame to either denounce or protect the surgeon. Only days after Luis Carlos was placed under house arrest, the Jalisco state governor, Emilio González Márquez, was asked to account for what had occurred. In an interview on 10 July in *Informador*, González Márquez sought to protect the reputation of the hospi-tal, but also his own, as he was officially responsible for signing off on the appoint-ment of staff at the hospital.

His response to any charge of illegality was to offer reassurance that any wrong-doing would be dealt with without prejudice to the hospital. Incidents such as these, he pointed out, do happen at institutions, but that does not necessarily lead to the institution in question. He strictly separated the event and the hospital, stat-ing that none of his managers needed to be questioned, as their principle con-cern was the effective running of the hospital. When it came to assigning blame, he suggested that those directly responsible ought to pay for what they did, with-out compromising the quality and prestige of the institution.[4]

His response shows transplant medicine to operate in ways similar to what Goffman (1961) described as a "workshop complex." Social institutions like hos-pitals are places where clients come to avail of specialist services, but where the routine work of those services is performed out-of-sight, away from public scru-tiny, where mistakes or alternative ways of getting the job done can be hidden from view. Scandals inevitably draw back the screen to reveal what happens behind it, opening actions to external scrutiny and judgement.

Distinguishing between the event and the institution would prove to be a major challenge for those wanting to protect the hospital's reputation. One route to tackling the problem was to mount a "bad apple" defense, an analytical strategy eagerly taken up in newspaper reports that directed attention to the infractions of the surgeon.[5] Efforts to separate out and distance other institutional actors from the surgeon highlighted the capacities of those with power to close ranks and externalize the problem, treating it as an aberration outside the domain of normal operations and thus not an official act at all. Doing so made it difficult to establish who knew what, thus creating a space for institutional deniability.

An interview for the magazine *Proceso* (Resa 2008) bears this out. In it, Jorge Enrique Segura Ortega, head of the Hepatology Department at Hospital Civil and ex rector of the University of Guadalajara's health and life sciences campus, suggested that both Leobardo Alcalá Padilla and Jaime Augustin González Álvarez, former directors of the public hospital, had been aware that Rodríguez Sancho was charging up to one million pesos for organ transplants. In addition to this, he drew attention to what he referred to as the indifference of the previous health secretary and now mayor of Guadalajara, Alfonso Petersen and the current health secretary, Alfonso Gutierrez, to the issue.

Ortega had much to gain from distancing himself from the work of the surgeon. In 1999, he had invited Rodríguez Sancho to be part of the team to implement a transplant program but later, he stated, as rumors of illicit charging for organs started to circulate, he stepped back from the project. He suggested that if the previous hospital management said they didn't know about the irregular charging, they were lying, and that the surgeon himself had confirmed that hospital authorities knew about the charges. Sancho remarked that the success of the transplant program had become so important to the city and the country that it had become a political instrument used to pressurize the authorities when required. All in all, Segura Ortega could not comment on the specifics of the allegations, whether there was any evidence of organ trafficking, or whether a crime had actually taken place, but asserted that any manipulation of organ waiting lists to favor those who could pay was a lamentable act of misconduct, particularly in the context of an institution established to respond to the needs of people who were uninsured. Those without economic means thus found themselves enrolled for various political ends and purposes.

Other detractors included Salvador Cosío Gaona who, as mentioned above, ran the NGO Conciencia Cívica Jalisciense. Through this organization, Cosío Gaona provided legal support for families wishing to take cases against the surgeon. At one press conference, reported in *Informador* (2008d), Cosío Gaona suggested that not only had the surgeon benefitted from unlawful transplant practices, so too had state officials, healthcare, and union leaders—a further extension of the behind-the-scenes workings of the local transplant project. He called into account the short period—effectively two days—of Rodríguez Sancho's house arrest. In response to Cosío Gaona's claims, the director of the Hospitales Civiles Trust, also in attendance at the press conference, suggested that Cosío Gaona's criticisms were nothing but a performance, an exercise in crude politicking rather than an expression of any real concerns over healthcare.

The press conference was, in many respects, an important forum for drawing attention to a much wider set of concerns associated with organ transplantation in the state; in particular, the perennial worry that those who were in a position to pay had privileged access, while others who were not simply died waiting. In this respect, misgivings and misunderstandings alike highlighted and brought to the surface the ways in which the local workings of transplant medicine generated public troubles around the transfer and allocation of organs. Juan Manuel Juarez Estrada of the Fundacion Nacional de Ninos Robados y Desaparecidos (National Foundation for Children, Taken and Disappeared) was also in attendance at the press conference and added further to these concerns. Juarez Estrada's fifteen-year-old son had died while he was waiting for a transplant. Estrada believed that the organ that had been donated to the boy by his uncle had gone to someone else.[6] Whether this was true or not, claims of foul play were portrayed as recurrent issues in a system fraught with perceptible inequalities. The alleged illegitimate practices, brought to attention by the scandal, offered few opportunities for resolution or change, but could at least be seen to provide a legitimate ground for airing grievances, worries, and concerns.

The surgeon's legal defense team contributed further to the problem of versions. They expended considerable efforts in a bid to ensure that the surgeon was seen as acting in good faith and that he was, if anything, the injured party. His actions, they argued, had been undertaken with the full knowledge of others. They pointed out that he could not possibly have acted alone. In an article in *Informador* (2008d), Juan Pablo Gudiño Coronado, Rodríguez Sancho's defense attorney, sought to show that responsibility did not lie with the surgeon, but with the hospital director Jaime Agustín González Álvarez. It was he who purportedly signed off on the surgeries, agreeing that they could take place, as long as the social work team means-tested the patients in question. Furthermore, Coronado suggested that there were a number of anomalies in the case against the surgeon, and he pointed out that the acceptance of private patients was not unusual and was permitted within private consultations, where patients did pay larger sums of money. Payments were assessed by the social work team at the hospital where patients were charged according to a means-tested scale. Coronado also stressed the benefit to the hospital in terms of fees accrued, which he proposed could be used to support free treatment for other patients.[7] He contended that if the intentions behind the accusations of wrongdoing on behalf of his client were political, they ought to be dealt with politically. If the intention was to discredit the surgeon, then this would affect the entire transplant team. Coronado was keen to note that among all of the complaints made against the surgeon, only the case of Xóchitl Armida Mestas Lomelí remained open. The other cases had been resolved in various ways through third-party negotiations.

REPERCUSSIONS

The transplant scandal brought to the surface a simmering political struggle within the higher ranks of the university administration and between this and the Hospitals' Trust. This led, among other things, to the rapid replacement of Briseño Torres as rector of the university. Attempts to broaden out questions of culpability beyond the surgeon and implicate the institution led to a decline in surgeries and in the public provision of deceased organs for transplant. This was widely publicized. From the point at which the scandal broke to when *La Contraloría* reached a verdict, only two transplants were carried out. Prior to that, the statistics, as reported, had been impressive, with 281 liver transplants and 490 kidney transplants performed in the previous ten years (*Informador* 2008d).

La Contraloría, the institution responsible for monitoring, regulating, and disciplining public servants, in the end issued a verdict. It suspended Rodríguez Sancho for a period of three years from working at the hospital and ordered him to repay 145,000 pesos (12,900 U.S. dollars). La Contraloría found that responsibility for "administrative irregularities/anomalies" lay with the surgeon. These irregularities, however, were never clearly spelled out. The only aspect of the verdict that moved the focus away from the surgeon was a request that the hospital make improvements to the transplant program.

The suspension and request for repayment were the only sanctions the surgeon received, and the verdict brought events to a formal conclusion. Rodríguez Sancho retained his private clinical posts and was said by staff at the hospital to have moved to a private medical institution in a neighboring state. Opinion on whether the sanctions were fair was split. Marco Antonio Cortés Guardado, the new rector of the university—Briseño Torres's replacement—took a very different view on the matter than his predecessor. In his view, the sanctions were particularly harsh, but he emphasized his respect for the judgement of the comptroller and stressed that the transplant program would continue. He stated that it was in the public interest to have the surgeon and his talents back at the public hospital in the near future.

There were many attempts to justify the deeds of the surgeon. Some claimed that Mexico's distinct lack of transplant specialists may have contributed to the irregularities, in that this produced a medical system constantly under pressure, where doctors had to do their job by whatever means they could. Promises were, nonetheless, made by those in charge at the hospital to improve the organization and delivery of renal care as well as medical training. Proposals were also made to retain the services and skills of the surgeon in the hope he could resume his post after a period of time. This, however, did not happen.

THE ANALYTICS OF ALIGNMENT: WHAT CAN BE LEARNED

Accounting for a scandal, particularly through the mediated sense-making of others, can only ever produce partial understandings. The boundaries that mark out its terrain of action and implication are contested, making it difficult to account with any certainty the size, scale, scope, and even character of the activities that took place. Nevertheless, the play of public accounts shows us that the contours of the scandal traversed the boundaries between the state, market, and medicine, and thus provide some access to the socio-political arrangements that intersect the project of transplant medicine and the interferences those arrangements can generate.

As a result, we can say that the lines of demarcation laid down to establish the boundaries of this scandal were socially invested. They help us identify those with a stake in the operations of transplant medicine, who, as a result, populate and staff its wider operations. This includes state and non-state actors: medical authorities, healthcare professionals, legal bodies, NGOs, bureaucrats and directors of various city-wide institutions, journalists, patients and their families, and many more besides. Collectively, they gave the scandal shape through the outcomes of different trials of strength and ensured particular understandings, actions, and reprisals came to the fore while others were sidelined. We see, therefore, in this scandal, a rich site of contestation and conflict, but we also see who has to do what for whom and under what conditions, in order to produce the grounds upon which a medical program, such as this, can, ought, or ought not to operate. This means that transplant medicine (and arguably other medical specialties) is not a discrete institutional practice, but one anchored to political promise, public reputation, city governance, and the modernizing projects of the state (Crowley-Matoka 2016).

In elaborating the social infrastructures upon which organ transplantation depend, it is critically important to pay attention to the analytical work of the actors themselves. This not only helps us to see how the scandal is made sense of by others and how it is used for various ends and means, but also how critique is organized from within and, through it, how opportunities for justice and recrimination are established or become blunted in the process. One of the things this book as a whole shows is that it is not simply the ethnographer who is trying to understand the events-in-question. Making sense of things was also a key preoccupation of all those with a vested interest in the operations of organ transplantation—from state officials, institutional, and organizational actors through to wider publics, and most importantly the patients who depend on the state's capacities for support and care. The challenge for the ethnographer is how to cope with what Rose and Miller (2010) have termed, "the multiple 'problematics' of government," or put another way, "the articulated dreams, schemes, strategies and maneuvers of authorities that seek to shape the beliefs and conduct of others by acting upon their will, their circumstances or their environment" (271). The disruptive consequences of the scandal provide us with insight into how the "multiple problematics of government" are made visible, and how the state is made visible.

Scandals provide such access because they imply some sort of wrongdoing, some illegitimate, inappropriate, or unsanctioned activity. Here the state is most strongly invoked. One of the classic roles of the state is to define such activity and to establish jurisdictions of responsibility, accountability, and arbitration. However, rather than act as a discrete juristic form, what we see at work in this case is a range of operations through which decisions and responses to illegitimate behavior are played out. Those operations are undertaken across a range of different institutional sites. Though far from exhaustive, in the case of this scandal, they included the Contraloria del Estado de Jalisco, the Procuraduría General de Justicia de Jalisco, the Comisión Estatal de Derechos Humanos de Jalisco, and COFEPRIS—the Comisión Federal para la Proteccion contra Riesgos Sanitarios—in addition to the public institutions of medicine itself. This diffusion of responsibility tells us something about the state and its responsibilities for the health, welfare, and protections of its people, but we have to be careful in setting that out.

The state, a much-theorized concern in anthropology and across the social sciences, is characterized by different analytical orientations toward it. Among these, the state can be conceived of as an entity abstracted from or acting on its citizens, set apart from and above society, coterminous with nation and territory; an ideological construct that unifies; or a material and rational construct that organizes and regulates our conduct—this is Hobbes's "Leviathan," Nietzsche's "cold monster," Hegel's "ethical project." However, ways of fixing definition and specified purpose to the state have found a range of counterpoints in the work of ethnographers like Begoña Aretxaga (1997), James Ferguson (1994), Akhil Gupta (1995, 2012), James Scott (1998), and Navaro-Yashin (2002)—all of whom attempt, in one way or another, to rethink the state-society divide. They show the work and idea of the state to be outcomes of social practice, underpinned in different ways, in different sites and settings by specificity, as features of everyday, routine encounters, which are bound up with other institutional forms: family, economy, healthcare, welfare, and so on. These authors suggest that our particular taken-for-granted ways of talking about state practice—its "vertical-encompassing character" as Ferguson and Gupta (2002) describe it—are less a reflection of how things are "in reality," functionally speaking, than a product of complex infrastructural arrangements found at the intersections of state and society. Weber (1946), whose classic definition of the state—a human community that successfully claims the monopoly of the legitimate use of physical force within a given territory— was inclined to see the state less as something defined by its ends and functions but rather as a complex of social interactions organized and oriented to normative practice. This complex of social interactions is thrown into relief by the transplant scandal, showing state-society relations to be mutually implicative and co-sustaining.

As the transplant project shows, the implications of society-state operations can mean a transfer of the operations of government to other entities. This might not necessarily mean less government but simply that other modalities are at play, such as the new models of enterprise seen via the extensions of pharma markets, medical suppliers, private medical practice, and the growth of a charitable sector (see chapter 5). Understanding how these various infrastructures work in relationship to the state is not simply a matter of starting with an idea of infrastructure first and then finding out what people do; instead we have to look at what people are doing and see how those infrastructures are made visible, and trace the various connections and processes that come to count.

As an instance of this, I want to briefly focus on two related infrastructural processes that can be derived from paying attention to the practices of some of the more powerful governmental actors at the heart of the transplant scandal. I refer to these processes as (a) the "accumulation of mandates" and (b) a "failure of transitivity."

An accumulation of mandates or *cumul des mandates* is often thought of as a controversial practice because it rests on an individual holding multiple positions across institutions, so setting up potential conflicts of interest. This accumulation of mandates is common to administrative and political office in Mexico, as directorships of various kinds are often populated by the same people moving between and across institutions. This strengthens the capacity of these socio-political actors to leverage action or interfere with the process of accountability, to quell a rumor mill or apportion reprisal and recrimination. An accumulation of mandates can protect and discredit. It also allows powerful elites to close rank, when needed; in this case, to protect a medical institution and isolate responsibility to the actions of an individual (however lenient and short lived that may have been).

In turn, as we have seen in this case, it also produces a "failure of transitivity," showing us how and why wrongdoing in one jurisdiction may not necessarily carry over to another: why an instance of medical malpractice may or may not be criminalized; why repercussions for the surgeon did not apply to other clinical environments; and why they did not hold in the public hospital over time. In the final assessments of this scandal, the lines of responsibility became particularly diffuse and entangled. However much Rodríguez Sancho was the main protagonist, it is also clear that his actions did not stand alone. Nonetheless, the manner in which the scandal proceeded meant it was contained; that high profile social actors closed ranks and, in doing so, political power bases remained fully intact—the self-same power bases from which the scandal emerged. These outcomes are certainly not restricted to medicine; they simply show how the systemic and routine nature of institutional operations can provide within them all manner of opportunities for misconduct.

Precisely because the systemic and routine operations of the clinic produce opportunities for misconduct, the "extraordinary" and "ordinary" are more closely aligned than we might think. The ground of the ordinary is, in fact, the ground of the extraordinary. Nonetheless, extraordinary activities also function to render ordinary activities ordinary by removing or casting extraordinary activities outside of normal routine functions.

The scandal that emerged from the events at the public hospital provided a prism through which everyday forms of doing medicine and providing treatment could be normalized, even when they were implicated in the systematic impoverishment of patients. However, because these systemic practices are difficult to extract, individualize, and personalize, it can be much more difficult to see the harms that extend from their mundane functions, and to critically engage with them, despite the fact that it is necessary to do so. In reflecting on the previous chapters where I examined the everyday ways in which patients attempt to gain access to transplant medicine, the story told might be considered no less scandalous than that outlined in this chapter. However, it is equally and unfortunately all too mundane. The routine ways in which those who are already poor are made catastrophically poorer, as they strip themselves of all their resources to access a healthcare system that does not benefit them, recurs in the accounts of patients like Elena, Emilio, Gabriel, and all those others portrayed in this book.

These mundane controversies might be best approached as an instance of what the anthropologist Veena Das (2006, 1) calls "everyday violence," a violence that has entered "the recesses of the ordinary" and, therefore, is no longer remarkable. This form of violence does not interrupt life, it is bound up with it; it isn't the exception, it is the rule. This poses certain methodological problems. In exceptional forms of wrongdoing, which interrupt the ordinary, in the harms they produce, witnessing has a special authority. We see this clearly and graphically through the sustained attention of city and state newspapers to the transplant scandal. However, when faced with infrastructural harms rooted in the systemic and slow-working mechanisms of medical institutions, it is not entirely clear what a witnessing might involve or how it ought to be articulated.

Scandals cannot be taken at face value or treated, at least in terms of their standard presentations, as an unproblematic given. Any facts we might be tempted to cling to tend to disintegrate, or at least blur around the edges, when competing versions of what actually happened are presented to us. Scandals exist in their multiple tellings. They do, however, provide grist to the analytical mill. Their very public nature allows us as ethnographers to pay close attention to how others make sense of what has occurred and how they mobilize its contents for their own ends and means. At the same time, we can also look for what is not told, searching out counterpoints and silences—alternative accounts that are not articulated, ways of seeing that do not become the basis of political disputes and turf wars but are treated by all sides as simply the way things are.

How and why anyone draws attention to wrongdoing or harm is an intensely political concern. Tracking scandal, in other words, has immense value to anthropologists. But it has to be approached carefully. We cannot carelessly add another account to the pile. We have to ask ourselves what we are doing in keeping scandals alive. Unless we treat them as avenues to a better understanding of that which we seek to study, there is a danger that we join the ranks of entrepreneurs seeking to capitalize on them for our own gain, offering yet another dramatization. The question is, then, not how we should report scandal but what the telling of scandal by different people, in different positions at different times, allows us to see about the contexts in which standards of right and wrong are formulated, fixed in place, and put to all manner of use. The following and final chapter continues with the idea of "unexceptional" harms as an instance of political economy. It does so by moving backward from the problems associated with technological interventions—the substantive focus of this book—to focus, instead, on the particular medical condition out of which technological interventions, indeed organ transplantation itself, extends. The chapter addresses the rise and spread of chronic kidney disease via a contemporary variant of it—chronic kidney disease of unknown origin—and its distinctly complex etiology.

7 · POLITICAL AND CORPORATE ETIOLOGIES

Producing Disease Emergence and Disease Response

In a small village, nestled on the shores of picturesque Lake Chapala, live three generations of the Martinez family. This is a family afflicted by chronic kidney disease. David, the middle child of six children, was diagnosed with CKD in 2013 but died two months later. He was eighteen years old and the causes of his condition were unknown. Three years later, his older brother Eduardo was diagnosed with the same condition, and the causes were similarly unknown. David and Eduardo's mother, Lola, had been diagnosed four years before David's death, again without any explanation. Her own brother—David and Eduardo's uncle—was also diagnosed with kidney disease of unknown causes; so too was her niece Maria. Only Lola's uncle, an older man in his sixties, another kidney patient in the family, had been told that his kidney disease had resulted from hypertension.

One by one, members of the Martinez family were slowly, inextricably, and sometimes fatally entangled in regimes of renal care and made to answer all their demands and requirements. As this chapter will go on to discuss, transplant medicine, as the preferred biotechnical fix for CKD, is poorly equipped to respond to the alarming number of patients presenting with rapidly failing kidneys in places such as Mexico. Organ transplantation offers a compromised response to the range of causes that are increasingly associated with the rise and spread of the condition. Tracing the experiences of families like that of the Martinez, and drawing out lessons from previous chapters, I argue that transplant medicine, as it has come to be organized and made to work in Mexico, is often best seen as an expression of the problems that accompany CKD, rather than a solution to them. Because its modes of operation reflect and operate in line with the kinds of inequalities that also characterize the spread of CKD, transplant medicine works to amplify the problems suffered by poor people, even as it seeks to alleviate them. Even worse, in alleviating problems it creates more troubles still. What, then, are the prospects for kidney transplantation in Mexico? Will it flourish or retract? And at whose expense?

The intensification or clustering of kidney disease within the context of extended families as well as in impoverished social and environmental settings has become, in recent years, part of the changing narrative of kidney disease. Practically everyone I met while doing fieldwork could tell me something about the condition or had someone close to them suffering from it. Many of the researchers and healthcare professionals I worked with had their own personal stories. Some of the nephrology staff at Hospital Civil had specifically chosen the specialty because of personal experience. Kidney disease was ubiquitous in Jalisco. A condition that rarely affects multiple members of the same family in European or North American households, it was too often a shared experience here.

One of the distinguishing features of the storied character of CKD was whether a diagnosis of the condition revealed an established cause. With respect to the patients I encountered, older renal patients in their fifties and upward were told their condition was the result of diabetes, hypertension, genetic predisposition, or injury. They were provided with explanations. For those who were younger—teenagers and those in their early twenties (a demographic that features prominently in this book)—explanations were less forthcoming. Instead, young people would say they had *riñones chiquitos* or *riñones pequeños* (small kidneys), a term often used as a proxy explanation or cause. *Riñones chiquitos* usually meant one of two things: that the patient had been born with small kidneys—a congenital condition, otherwise known as renal hypoplasia, which can lead to CKD—*or* that their kidney disease was advanced prior to diagnosis, and this had resulted in a scarring or shrinkage of the organ, such that it was difficult to perform an effective biopsy to establish a cause. *Riñones chiquitos* has, in many respects, come to symbolize the challenges and problems of diagnosing what is today considered a new variant of chronic kidney disease, one that is steadily on the rise in Mexico.

CHRONIC KIDNEY DISEASE OF UNKNOWN ORIGIN

In this chapter I examine this new variant of chronic kidney disease, namely chronic kidney disease of unknown origin (CKDu), and its implications for understanding the limits and possibilities of regimes of renal care. CKDu has been variously linked to instances of state, corporate, and environmental harm, with reference to, among other things, the effects of a heavily processed food industry, poor toxic waste management, unchecked use of pesticides, and contaminated water. It is a condition that positions the body not only as the site where disease finds expression, but where the state, market, and medicine meet in highly variable and disruptive ways. CKDu and the biotechnical responses that have grown around it—the subject of this book thus far—are intimately connected as cause, effect, and care, all similarly shaped by the same social and political conditions.

In order to give these social and political conditions proper consideration and bring structure to the account that follows, I treat CKDu as a worksite, one around which different types of social actors coalesce to produce new insights, understandings, and interventions. As a worksite, CKDu represents a rich ground of communicability in at least two senses. First, following Holmes (2013), facts about the world begin by being worked up in communicative fields—akin to Shapin and Schaffer's discursive technologies discussed in chapter 1—prior to their becoming empirical givens. Diagnostic categories are not neutral but reflect the social and political processes and inequities that go into making and stabilizing them (Briggs and Mantini-Briggs 2016; Latour 1987). Second, drawing on Seeberg and Meinert (2015), chronic conditions such as diabetes, depression, eating disorders, and kidney disease should be understood as the outcome of communicable forces in their rise, spread, and epidemic potential. Seeberg and Meinert contend that "communicability," as a term that often distinguishes and divides chronic from infectious diseases (i.e., communicable versus non-communicable), has been poorly conceptualized, misleading the construction and understanding of contemporary epidemics. Rethinking the nature of communicability attunes us to the social and political economic forces that shape CKDu's emergence and its capacity to spread in specific environments. In the context of Mexico, this can take into consideration the legacy of NAFTA, the effect of trade agreements that have seen indigenous industry, labor rights, environmental integrity, and food safety suffer, while multi- and transnational corporations enjoy an incentivized and deregulated market for their goods. How this affects the health and wellbeing of Mexico's citizens has barely begun to be calculated, as attempts to account for CKDu show.

CKDu is a major public health concern across countries of the global south, notably in Central America and Southeast Asia. The WHO standardized the use of the category in 2008, in consideration of the escalation of the condition in Sri Lanka. Although systems of reporting and surveillance are partial, if not altogether lacking, across countries, the condition can be traced back at least four decades to Central America, according to research conducted among sugar cane workers in Guanacaste, Costa Rica (Trabanino et al. 2002; Wesseling et al. 2015). As early as 1978, men living and working in Guanacaste were reported to be twice as likely to develop an unexplained variant of CKD than the average Costa Rican male, with those cutting sugar cane more than four times more likely.

CKDu, since then, has grown in its associations with impoverished communities, poor and stressful working conditions (particularly for agri-working men), degraded environments and exposures to toxins and heavy metals. According to the Pan American Health Organization (PAHO 2014), hospitalizations for CKD in agricultural communities in Central America increased by 50 percent from 2005 to 2012, and the condition is now the leading cause of hospital deaths. In El

Salvador and Nicaragua, where sugar cane production dominates agricultural work, CKDu or MeN (Mesoamerican nephropathy—another acronym used to denote its disproportionate effect on men in the region) has emerged as a perilous problem for those aged between fifteen and forty-nine years in these countries. El Salvador and Nicaragua have, respectively, the first and second highest probabilities of dying of kidney disease anywhere in the world.

CKDu is a vexing challenge in the field of global health. Documenting its rise and spread has become a critical imperative. While epidemiological research has started to map the emergence of CKDu across sub-Saharan Africa, parts of India, Nepal, China, Sri Lanka, and the Middle East, in addition to Central America, it is not always apparent that what presents as CKDu in one place is the same as in another or, indeed, whether the condition arises out of the same sets of social and economic conditions (Stanifer et al. 2016). MeN in Central America, for example, is widely hypothesized to be an outcome of consistent heat exposure and dehydration due to strenuous outdoor agri-work, such as in the case with sugar cane production (Wesseling, Crowe, and Hogstedt 2013). In Sri Lanka, while the rise of CKD has also been linked to the working conditions of agri-workers, what has attracted most attention has been the use of agrochemicals, polluted water, and the presence of heavy metals, in addition to heat stress and dehydration (de Silva, Albert, and Jayasekara 2017; WHO 2016).

The only part of the world where an identifiable cause has been attributed to the condition has been in the Balkan region. Classified as Balkan nephropathy, a sudden rise of CKD was reported across rural Bosnia, Bulgaria, Croatia, Romania, and Serbia as early as 1956, and in a more steady fashion during the 1970s and 1980s (Pavlović 2013). It was initially assumed that an environmental toxin was responsible, but nothing was found. A cluster of young Belgian women, all diagnosed with rapidly progressing CKD, provided some clues. They had been using a Chinese herbal remedy to aid weight loss, extracted from the Aristolochia plant.[1] Its central ingredient, aristolochic acid, is a known nephrotoxin (Martín-Cleary and Ortiz 2014). The plant, endemic to the Balkans, was often mixed with wheat to make bread, thereby providing an unambiguous culprit (Grollman, Scarborough, and Jelaković 2009). Balkan nephropathy, however, is singular and anomalous in the causal story of CKDu, unrepresentative of what is thought to be happening elsewhere.

CKDu, as its classification suggests, resists standard explanations. No one discipline has been able to claim epistemic authority over it, and it is doubtful if this could be possible given its elusive, contextually variable character. Part of the problem lies in the persistent challenge of producing reliable and comparative epidemiological data adequate to a condition of this kind. There are, to date, few studies advancing a comprehensive account of the nature, distribution and spread of the condition in its variant forms, and those that exist are wrought with difficulties as to how best to report and assess it.

What we do know is that CKDu is categorically different to CKD. As stated in the introduction, both conditions are similarly degenerative and progressive, but marked by different determinants. CKD is the outcome of conditions such as, diabetes, glomerulonephritis, polycystic kidney disease, vascular disease, genetic disorders, congenital problems, and injury, among others, all of which tell their own articulated and extended etiological stories. CKDu, in contrast, is predominantly associated with working and living in poor agricultural settings, often in hot climates. Patients with CKD present with glomerular damage accompanied by the existence of proteins in their urine; those with CKDu present with glomerular and tubular damage, but do not exhibit proteins until the condition is far advanced. The common approach for establishing a diagnosis of CKD is by measuring the glomerular filtration rate (GFR) and levels of proteins in urine—both, however, are limited in terms of sensitivity and specificity for CKDu, and are therefore weak diagnostic markers. As Stanifer and colleagues (2016) point out, for low- and middle-income countries (LMICs) , in particular, validated creatinine-based tests for estimating glomerular filtration rate or standardized, quality-controlled measurements of serum creatinine or urinary protein are simply not available.[2]

As stated before, the causes of CKDu are complicated by the fact that the kidneys are often so atrophied that they are impossible to biopsy, providing little traction for understanding. The biopsy, nevertheless, remains a gold standard for diagnosing kidney disease. Even when the kidneys are amenable to it, it is an invasive procedure that requires highly qualified experts for its performance and interpretation, skills that are not always available in the places in which CKDu emerges (Levin et al. 2017). Further still, for Mexico, in a fragmented healthcare system where patient data is not easily shared, where public health monitoring is partial, where dialysis and transplant registry data have poor coverage, and where the patients who suffer most from failing kidneys fall outside state systems of monitoring, welfare, and entitlement, there are limits in ascertaining the percentage of CKD deaths that can actually be classified as CKDu.

What is also clear is that understanding the scale of the problem and the interacting causal chains that produce it are impossible when using the tools of a single disciplinary perspective. Having confidence that what appears to be CKDu is in fact CKDu is far from straightforward, making attempts to isolate it for the purposes of analysis an epistemologically treacherous affair. In 2016, when I first mentioned to one of my nephrology participants that I was interested in developing a new research project to document the lives of patients with CKD of unknown etiology, I was told explicitly that no cases had yet been identified in Mexico, and that what was occurring was unlike what had been reported in Central America. One year later, the nephrologist in question was raising his own concerns about the emergence of CKDu at international conferences, in line with other medical teams across the global south.

The reluctance of my nephrology colleague to claim CKDu as a problem is not surprising, nor is it a limitation of his insight, imagination, or observational skills. CKDu is a classificatory problem in addition to being an empirical one (Bowker and Star 1999; Hacking 2006). How this classification comes to be stabilized and articulated by others is as much a social as a bioscientific process. Establishing that CKDu exists in Mexico is limited not only by a general lack of related population statistics and the variable diagnostic techniques used to identify the condition, but also because those diagnostic techniques are hampered by the fact that many patients often present so late to doctors. Producing data that can be reliably compared across settings is compounded by the variable conditions in which CKDu emerges, and by the fact that information sharing between medical institutions is not made particularly easy in a highly fragmented healthcare system. Added to this is, of course, the fact that formally recognizing CKDu as a problem requires political will, which, in turn, necessitates some form of action. Given what we already know from the previous chapters about the profound challenges facing those who are attempting to access renal care, and those who are attempting to provide it, this new variant of CKD will create untold pressures on an already stressed healthcare system, the implications of which have not gone unnoticed (Wesseling, Crowe, and Hogstedt 2013).

In a context where the disclosure of a major new public health problem would create political problems due to public demands for intervention, it is in the interest of governors to play the role of skeptic and ask for evidence. Such requests often translate into unattainable levels of certainty. In the absence of any capacity to produce such certainties, efforts to account for or raise awareness about CKDu have been driven by a wide array of forces both within and outside the medical domain. These include the many efforts of community and environmental activists, epidemiologists, public health researchers, toxicologists, journalists, and more, as well as government officials and politicians. All have entered into the debate at different moments in time, from different perspectives, with different issues at stake and with often vastly different methods and systems for generating an understanding of what is or might be happening. CKDu not only speaks in a confusion of tongues; it has become an intensely political controversy contested outside formal political arenas via a play of differentially leveraged claims and counterclaims by stakeholders with profoundly varying political capacities. My work is no different; it too is situated within, takes its lead from, and constitutes a move within this controversy. Via the fieldwork that forms the basis of my research, CKDu made itself known at the precarious intersections of poverty, work, and the environment, a distinct expression of a "local biology" (Lock 2001), an outcome of geographical, geological, historical, political, economic, social, and pathophysiological processes. These intersections are a way of attending to CKDu, as well as to the many other investigators who have also converged at this worksite.

The Martinez family are the living embodiment of what emerges when we attend to these intersecting domains. Like the other families who live in their small lakeside village, precarity underscores the everyday working and domestic practices of their household. The Martinez family live in a continual state of intergenerational flux. Often three to four generations are present at any one time, sometimes to share meals and sometimes to share accommodation, as the needs and circumstances of working life demand and allow. The household is, as a result, improvised and haphazard. It is very often overcrowded, with little by way of personal space, making it especially challenging to live with sickness and care for a loved one who is enduring the end stages of kidney functioning on home dialysis or recovering from transplant surgery. In the absence of welfare entitlements, the labor required to support kidney disease financially and morally, as discussed in previous chapters, is widely distributed among family members. Everyone also works, yet it is not easy to establish what the precise nature of each family member's employment status is. Across three generations of grandparents, parents, and teenage children, members of the family have variously found work as contract laborers with the local transnational berry companies, as construction workers on building projects in Guadalajara, on local farms, in the local fishing industry, as domestic cleaners in nearby towns, and as cultivators of crops on their own small landholdings or gardens. Work is variable, impermanent and, at times, in relation to health, harmful. Children, too, contribute to the daily round of domestic tasks, gathering sticks for cooking, picking, and selling fruit and vegetables, spraying agrochemicals on family land holdings, and helping out as and when needed.

The Martinez family is poor. They collectively function as an economic unit, living precariously within the country's growing informal economy, living without adequate state supports. Their diets are also poor, comprising a staple of corn and beans, fish from the lake, and whatever can be grown or domesticated in their households or small holdings. They are reliant on improvised cooking facilities, largely homemade wood-burning stoves, which operate throughout the day in poorly ventilated spaces—these stoves are heavily implicated in the rise of pulmonary conditions like chronic obstructive pulmonary disorder (COPD). The lived environment that surrounds the Martinez family is fragile. Lake Chapala, a major concern for environmental activists, is reputed to be highly contaminated with heavy metals, if not outright toxic, yet it is central to the everyday lives of those whose homes are dotted along its shorelines. The lake is a place to bathe, wash clothes and household items, catch fish, and draw water (see figure 8). In the absence of a local refuse service in the Martinez's village, the edge of the lake also serves as a site for waste disposal. The lake edge is where many household gardens end, and it functions as the preferred place to burn household rubbish, the remnants of which are carried away by the lake's waters. CKD is, of course, not the only affliction to be endured here: malnutrition, congenital

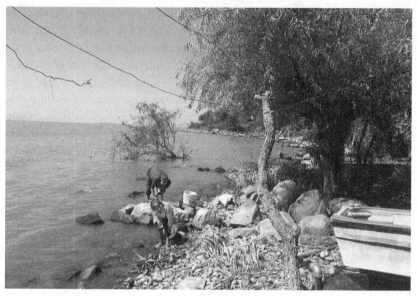

FIGURE 8. Lake Chapala.

physical malformations, poor cognitive development, cancers, alcoholism, diabetes, among other conditions, compete for attention, resources, publicity, and political commitment. All of these problems are made worse still by difficulties in accessing doctors, dentists, pharmacies, midwives, and so on. For the young people who have been identified as especially vulnerable to CKDu, their need for appropriate and timely healthcare is critical but structurally unattainable.

CKD of unknown origin, as it emerges in the context of Lake Chapala, discloses and throws into relief the relationship between a troubled environment and the wellbeing of the people who live there. Land and soil, lake and water, food and ways of working; an entire living ecology and ecology of living, are shown to be enduringly fragile and wrought with debilitating risk. The landscape of Chapala is not an unobtrusive background to everyday life, concealing its own significance, diverting attention from influence. It is very visibly in the foreground—a provocation (Hastrup 2016), an event of configuration (Massey 2005), something that commands attention whenever life around the lake is examined. One reason the landscape forces itself upon us is because it lays bare its own histories and constitutive logics and the forms of life they afford, by distilling global networks and shifting assemblages of progress, bringing together capital, waste and land exploitation, precarity and vulnerability (Gordillo 2014).

The landscape of Chapala—its soil and water—points to an uncertain future for those who live there. It shows that growth as the calculus of human development constitutes the terms by which we understand health and harm. As Anna Tsing (2015) notes, our assumption of the trope of progress is that it is sufficient to know the world, in its successes and failures. Progress, she suggests, still controls us, even in tales of ruination: "We are stuck with the problem of living despite economic and ecological ruination. Neither talk of progress nor ruin tells us how to think about collaborative survival" (Tsing 2015, 19). The challenge of collaborative survival is the perplexing problem for the people who live by the lake, as well as for those with a stake in their health and welfare. How to do so in the context of a problem we don't yet understand requires what Tsing refers to as the "art of noticing," noticing what happens at the unruly edges where nature and culture, environment, and society cannot so easily be divided and made to stand apart. To acquire an understanding of CKDu, "noticing" has become critical.

What might the art of noticing involve when the object of interest is categorically "unknown"? CKDu is not a category that can speak for itself; there is nothing evident about what can or cannot be said about it or what might be possible to do with it. Neither does CKDu denote an absence of knowledge, nor a state of blind ignorance. CKDu is a "known unknown"; its content and infrastructure are yet to be specified and catalogued (Nielsen and Sørensen 2015). It signifies knowledge that has not yet been settled, marking out a terrain of hypotheses, disputes, contests, and vested interests, where potential knowledge makers contribute to the production of claims and counter claims cast in their own image (Fujimura and Chou 1994).[3] CKDu has the status of a fully fledged "scientific controversy," and so takes its place among prior biomedical controversies that serve as sensitizing precedents, as illustrated by the case of syphilis (Fleck 1979 [1935]) and by Latour (1987) on the relationship between microbes and disease. That CKDu retains an ambiguous ontology underscores the multiple interests and politics converging on the condition, some attempting to make it disappear, others to make it more visible, but none adequate to alter either position, none able to achieve epistemic authority.

Across the global south, a growing international community has coalesced around this complex condition representing different disciplinary interests, modes of problematization, methodological orientations, and efforts at explanation. Examples of such work in Latin America can be seen via The Consortium for the Epidemic of Nephropathy in Central America and Mexico (CENCAM) and La Isla Foundation and its associated multi-stakeholder initiatives, such as The Worker Health and Efficiency (WE) Program and the Adelante Initiative.[4] Nevertheless, the production of scientific knowledge around CKDu or MeN, particularly via peer-reviewed academic papers, is still very much in its infancy.

The picture is somewhat different when one scales down into the localities where CKDu is causing alarm. In the communities of Chapala, where the Martinez family live, concerns about kidney failure have intensified, particularly in the last decade.[5] Within these local contexts we see a picture of CKDu emerge through the efforts of those who live and work there, assembled by the differently motivated efforts of local families and citizens, environmental, health activists and researchers, journalists, doctors, epidemiologists, toxicologists, religious and civil society organizations, and government officials. Sometimes operating as allies, sometimes as adversaries, their collective responses have turned CKDu and the communities it is understood to afflict into "worksites." This has served to produce not only knowledge, but also the skeptical anxieties and counter-strategies that help to maintain this variant of kidney disease in its epistemological limbo.

CKDU AS WORKSITE

Taking forward the idea of CKDu as a worksite, I focus briefly on some of the social actors who have been and continue to be central to producing understandings and awareness of this condition and whose efforts exemplify the pivotal intersections between activism, medicine, and bioscientific research.

I start with Jorge, a religious man so moved by compassion for those living in sickness and poverty around Chapala Lake that he has embarked on a personal mission to support their efforts to access healthcare. He transports patients without means to and from medical appointments. For those on hemodialysis, their weekly regimen has now become his. He is particularly sensitive to what he has personally witnessed as an increase in CKD among young people, as well as the disproportionate presence of congenital physical disabilities among the lakeside communities. Along with other concerned citizens living in the area, he attributes the rise of chronic diseases to the polluted lake and to concerns over heavy metals found in tap water and local wells.[6] Charged by the conviction that responding to the needs of the poor and sick was his calling to do God's work, he has gone to extraordinary lengths to document, publicize, and politicize the health problems experienced by those living by Chapala Lake. He has painstakingly gathered information on water contamination, has made his own registries of patients with kidney disease, organized public meetings, academic workshops, and public demonstrations. He has drawn into conversation doctors, researchers, journalists, and politicians—anyone who he considers of relevance to the issue, who might listen, and who might be able to intervene. Such are the extent of Jorge's connections that one has only to follow his work in order to find out who else is working on or concerned with CKDu.

Jorge's particular mode of health evangelism was emboldened by Pope Francis's (2015) papal encyclical *Laudato Si* ("Praised Be"), which was a central aspect of the Pope's visit to Latin America that same year. In it, Pope Francis described climate change as the great moral issue of our time, while decrying the excesses of industrialization and the destruction of the natural environment. Jorge's efforts to help by raising awareness about well and lake water and, most particularly, this new and emerging form of kidney disease, have, however, polarized others similarly interested in and committed to addressing the problem. While some of the medical community have enrolled his efforts, using his proximity to the community as well as the data he has amassed, to supplement their own knowledge and understanding, others consider him to be cavalier, concerned that his politicizing of the condition interferes with the more tentative and cautious steps taken as part of careful research practice. Others still have raised concerns that his ardent focus on water as the sole source of contamination might actually serve to downplay wider structural problems of poverty, in particular the precarious nature of agricultural work and lives lived in poorly resourced and underserved communities.

From the perspective of those most central to the medical care of kidney patients, in particular those working in nephrology, the growing concerns about CKDu in the region have generated ambivalences. Medical staff are in little doubt that they are experiencing a rise in patients presenting with an unexplained form of CKD, many in relatively advanced stages, and among a younger demographic. However, as one nephrologist made clear, attempts to deal with the already existing demands for renal replacement therapies have stretched many hospitals and clinics to the limits of their resources. How to accommodate the, as yet, unpredictable challenge of the rise and spread of CKDu is a problem that has to be met in measured terms: professional competences, institutional reputations, and the patients themselves need to be protected. CKDu presents renal medicine with a conundrum. To identify and draw attention to a new healthcare crisis, a potential epidemic—one that no one understands—without the capacity to treat it or stop it, could create a parallel crisis of trust in a healthcare system that is already under pressure. As my nephrology colleague explained, "it is very important that our patients are reassured that everything that can be done, is being done."

The politics of healthcare resourcing and the pressures on health professionals to navigate the sensitive terrain between their own medical institutions, their patients, and the government bodies that support them, shape what can and cannot be said about CKDu. For a nephrologist, any desire to raise awareness of the condition is undermined by uncertainties as to whether or not Mexican healthcare is witnessing the same type of phenomenon seen in Nicaragua and El Salvador, particularly when screening and diagnostic procedures are not adequate to need. What comes to count as a new biomedical category is not only contingent on a politics of evidence, but also on a political economy of healthcare provision that designates what can and cannot be treated. What is particularly important in coming to an understanding of a complex concern like CKDu are the ways in which disease etiology, disease expression, and medical response—cause, effect, and care—are themselves intimately connected, shaped by but also serving to shape, society, morality, and politics. As writing in the field of science studies has shown, knowledge and intervention, problem definition and proposed solution, very often reflect and are modulated by one another not once and for all, but in ongoing ways (Fujimura and Chou 1994).

CKDu as a worksite will continue to give rise to further modulations as the configurations of interested parties organized around and through it continue to shift and change. The directions those shifts and changes might take are partially detectable in the stances those working on the problem take with respect to others. Outside of the provision of medical care, a team of epidemiological and biosci-entific researchers have in similar ways but for different reasons exercised caution in responding to the claims of water activists and the work of Jorge. Over the past two to three years, these researchers, working in the locality on a cluster of envi-ronmental health projects, have examined increases in cases of renal damage, among other conditions, within what are thought of as hot spots around Chapala Lake. Their work has generated a range of hypotheses, extending from the pres-ence of heavy metals found in blood and urine samples, to the use of agrochemi-cals, to impoverished diet, poor nutrition, and genetic factors, in addition to the possible contamination of lake water. The approach they have taken at this early stage is to avoid jumping to conclusions too quickly and instead they have taken a longer view—operating a "multiple causes–multiple effects" approach to under-standing sickness in the context of the lake, poverty, and perceived environmen-tal damage. As a consequence, the researchers have been careful not to become overly identified with activist research in general and Jorge in particular.

While skeptical about the role of lake water as a cause of CKDu, the principal researcher leading one of these projects was also careful not to deny that the water could be a source of contamination. To do so might imply he was acting as a con-duit for local politicians, who declare the lake water to be safe and defend the work of their municipalities to maintain clean and functioning water systems. Nev-ertheless, the researcher in question regularly pointed out that because CKDu appeared to disproportionately affect women more than men in the communi-ties in which he was working, the lake water was unlikely to be the cause—he jus-tified his claim on the basis that he did not know of any water system that might discriminate on the basis of gender, but also ignored the different ways in which women and men might be exposed to water. Nevertheless, the idea of "bad water" retains persuasive force in the public imagination and is unlikely to be easily dis-lodged. Given that there are very few formally funded studies of the complex causes of sickness among lakeside communities, and certainly less on CKDu, those currently generating knowledge of the issue are routinely and actively engaged in forms of boundary making to establish what may or may not count as legitimate claims with respect to the condition. The tensions that arise and char-acterize the relationships between patients, activists, healthcare professionals, sci-entists, and politicians produce communicative inequities, which, in turn, extend and deepen health inequities (Briggs and Mantini-Briggs 2016). Nading and Lowe (2018), writing on the epidemic control of CKDu and the Zika virus, character-ize these inequities as a problem of "representative justice," a form of social jus-tice that emphasizes the recognition and representation, not only of experienced medical problems, but of the entangled histories of racial, gendered, and economic inequity of which they are apart. These communicative inequities are keenly felt

in the everyday arbitrations to settle whose versions of CKDu count. This rudi-
mentary and rather crude sketch of CKDu, as it has emerged around Chapala
Lake, indicates some of the contingencies that frame an emergent local debate and
how different forms of knowledge come to count or acquire expedience. The subject of "bad water" serves as a reminder that when a problem such as this is
viewed from the perspective of a religious activist, a medical doctor, or an epidemiologist, very different concerns are at stake. Jorge, for example, is not engaged
in his activism because he wants to construct scientific knowledge claims, which
may well be the case for the researcher and the doctor; rather, he wants to fulfil
his moral duty as a Christian, and that is to alleviate suffering. Similar considerations arise around the work of researchers and doctors too. For these reasons,
attempts to build a picture of a phenomenon like CKDu are as contextually sensitive as the condition itself appears to be. The avenues of explanation that any
interested party might pursue and advance reflect their commitments and are an
outcome of training, values, and world views, coupled with their specific engagements and experiences with the problem. It is these practices and perspectives
within which the category "unknown" acquires content. It is far from surprising
that nephrologists will medicalize CKDu, that activists will politicize or moral-
ize it, that journalists will sensationalize it, and politicians will suppress or advance
it depending on what might be deemed to be at stake politically in affirming or
denying its existence. An understanding of CKDu is slowly taking shape through
the unpredictable alliances and collaborations it fosters as a shared worksite where
the question of how to do the required work is endlessly revisited and disputed.

While these various stakeholders interact with each other regularly, alliances
between them are fragile—particularly in a context where activists want upstream
solutions and doctors need to demonstrate them further downstream. A character like Jorge, nevertheless, is particularly interesting. He is an important inter-
locutor, one who is crucial to follow and who will raise the contentious issues that
no one else will. In this, he is like Becker's "moral outsider" or Shapin and Schaffer's "scandalous figure," whose significance it is easy to overlook in the final analysis precisely because he seems eccentric, peripheral, and unruly. One of the
strengths of his position, however, is that the concerns he raises are real—real in
the consequences they have for poor communities living around Chapala Lake—
even if the explanations he posits are not (or at least not yet).

RETHINKING THE STRUCTURAL BASE

There is much work to be done in generating explanations of CKDu, but that does
not mean that there are not pragmatic places to begin. It is certainly possible to
understand the conditions within which this story gets told, what constitutes its
central features and who is recruited into or ostracized by the communicative practices that ground it. In interrogating CKDu, we are interrogating "cultures in

contention" (Haraway 1989) that drive the production and processes of medical knowledge making. The capacity of such cultures to create both "truth" spots and "blind" spots open up as they close down different avenues of inquiry: land use, environmental harm, labor conditions, use of pesticides, the disposal of waste, poor access to safe food and water, and so on. Taken together they are, in the broadest sense, communicable features, whose practices and affects have much to teach us about what is happening when chronic diseases spread, when they become entangled in new processes of contagion (Whyte 2012)—processes that are the outcome of political economy (Adams 2016; Biehl and Petryna 2013).

How precisely to understand the role of political economy in shaping disease outcomes remains a persistent challenge to research, policy, and practitioner communities. Seeberg and Meinert (2015) remark that despite recognition of the significance of political and structural forces in the rise and emergence of chronic conditions worldwide, they continue to be cached out in terms of behavior and lifestyle.[7] They note that while the WHO suggests that major reductions in the burden of non-communicable diseases ought to come from population-wide structural interventions, these are not implemented due to inadequate political commitment. Instead, the WHO continues to espouse a focus on healthy lifestyles as the single most important preventive strategy (Seeberg and Meinert 2015).

The failure to accommodate the structural features of disease emergence within a discourse of prevention and intervention urges a look back in time at the "epidemiological transition," that which broadly signaled a break with persistent infectious diseases as a result of interventions in sanitation, sewerage, and the provision of clean water.[8] Writing over 150 years ago, Rudolf Virchow, the German pathologist, notable for his work on the typhus epidemic in what was then Upper Silesia (now Poland), shifted focus from the bacterial or animal vectors that transmit typhus to humans to argue for the social, economic, and cultural factors that he saw as responsible for the epidemic in the first place, for example, a lack of employment, decent housing, education, and a safe environment. The capacity to see public health in such terms today is not without its challenges. It is not easy to articulate the role of social, cultural, and political economic factors when the infrastructures they are bound to are increasingly transnational in character and where poor and precarious communities and workforces have few resources at their disposal to be heard—such as the power of collective action—to challenge the global forces that lay claim to their land, their livelihoods, and their health. In Mexico, we might look to NAFTA as a pertinent example of a transnational infrastructure implicated in the deterioration of a public's health. Alyshia Gálvez (2018) discusses the effects of NAFTA's elimination of subsidies that once helped Mexican agricultural producers to grow food, now replaced by the large-scale corporate North American producers who have flooded the Mexican market with industrially produced agrigoods. In the years following the signing of the NAFTA treaty, Mexico has seen a rise in chronic non-communicable diseases—

diabetes, heart disease, and CKD. The loss of life incurred contrasts to the wins of the U.S. food and beverage companies, which have saturated the Mexican market. Gálvez's research documents what she refers to as the "nutrition transition," namely when countries of the global south open their borders to global trade, they do so to the detriment of the public health of their citizens.[9] By allowing more foreign direct investment, trade and industrialization on an under-regulated basis, countries increase the risk of chronic disease for their citizens.

The vulnerability of sickness and disease to the macroparasites of the global market is a concern of many working in the field of global health today (Baer, Singer, and Susser 2003). For anthropologists, no matter how situated and local the phenomena we study, it is now more critical than ever to understand the rise, spread, and treatment of disease within the context of wider structural and infrastructural forces. In writing about the recent Ebola outbreak after his return from Liberia, Paul Farmer focused attention on the role of infrastructural harm in the epidemic. He explains:

> But the fact is that weak health systems, not unprecedented virulence or a previously unknown mode of transmission, are to blame for Ebola's rapid spread. Weak health systems are also to blame for the high case-fatality rates in the current pandemic, which is caused by the Zaire strain of the virus. The obverse of this fact—and it is a fact—is the welcome news that the spread of the disease can be stopped by linking better infection control (to protect the uninfected) to improved clinical care (to save the afflicted). An Ebola diagnosis need not be a death sentence . . . Ebola is more a symptom of a weak healthcare system than anything else. (2014, 38)

For Farmer, it was not the eating of bush meat, a widely reported cause of the virus, but the "grotesque and growing disparities in access to care—in the context of a globalized political economy" that led to the Ebola crisis (Farmer 2014, 38).[10] However, important as Farmer's work has been to shifting understandings of the etiology away from behavioral models and discrete causal chains of infection and toward the structural and political, there is room for greater specificity. Also writing in the aftermath of Ebola, Wallace and Wallace attempt to provide just that.[11] Describing disease epidemics as much markers of modern civilization as threats to it, they show how patterns of agri-economic exploitation raise the risk of epidemics in the first place, by detailing the specific ways in which intensive agriculture's diseconomies of scale degrade the resilience of ecosystems to disease. This accelerates pathogen spread and evolution by giving rise to genetic monocultures, high population densities, and expanding exports (Wallace and Wallace 2016). By way of example:

> For most of its history . . . Vibrio cholerae lived off plankton in the Ganges delta. It was only after significant layers of the population had switched to an urban,

sedentary lifestyle, and later had become increasingly integrated by nineteenth-century trade and transport systems, that the cholera bacterium evolved an explosive, human-specific ecotype. Simian immunodeficiency viruses emerged out of their non-human *Catarrhini* reservoirs in the form of HIV when colonial expropriation turned subsistence bushmeat and the urban sex trade into commodities on an industrial scale. Domesticated livestock has supplied a source for human diphtheria, influenza, measles, mumps, plague, pertussis, rotavirus A, tuberculosis, sleeping sickness and visceral leishmaniasis. Ecological changes wrought upon landscapes by human intervention have facilitated spillovers of malaria from birds, and of dengue and yellow fever from wild primates. (Wallace and Wallace 2016, 1)

When innovations in agricultural and industrial methods, alongside significant demographic shifts are seen in the context of poverty and inadequately resourced healthcare, a cascade of logistical failures follow—much as we have seen throughout this book in the case of CKD in Mexico. This amplifies transmission as a biosocial concern. Wallace and Wallace (2016) make clear that understanding pathogenic contexts and structural forces means much more than providing a background against which disease emergence can be set. These are not merely frames for generating understandings; rather, they are ways of identifying the specific processes (industrial, agricultural, political)—as well as the connections between them—that are implicated in the rise and spread of disease. In understanding these features of political economy as structural, we are able to see them as local work. In other words, by paying attention to the particularities of local arrangements, practices, and connections, the structural context is made available. Furthermore, in following these local connections, we may learn something vital about strategies for prevention and intervention, and the pertinent questions for researchers and practitioners in the twenty-first century (Wallace and Wallace 2016).

How to explore the local arrangements and forces implicated in the rise of CKDu and CKD is a significant challenge. There is undoubtedly a long road ahead. In this context, what does it mean to offer treatment and intervention? Can the biotechnical arrangements bound up with regimes of renal care offer sustainable solutions, or will their extensions exacerbate the disembedding of healthcare from social and collective responsibilities? In this case, both cause and cure, problem and solution, are entangled—both are expressions of the same processes and connections. The rise of CKDu suggests things are likely to get worse, not better, making the provision of renal care little more than a form of triage. The conditions in which transplant medicine seem likely to further flourish in Mexico are also conditions in which transplanted patients and their families will not.

CKDu emerges within what Anna Tsing (2005) refers to as a "zone of awkward engagement," one within which poverty and inequality, precarious work, unsafe living conditions, and the exploitation of land and water by global capital, throw into contention the competing forces of surplus accumulation (at national and transnational levels) with the basic necessities of getting by for the majority of Mexico's citizens. These forces represent "frictions," diverse and conflicting social interactions that make up our contemporary world and that generate its harms and excesses (Tsing 2005). It is certainly impossible to treat the effects of frictions until we understand the levels and scales upon which their harms are manifest— physiologically, phenomenologically, and politically. How to identify the connections that configure the enigma of CKDu is problematic when working from an imperfect knowledge base. However, as Holmes (2013) suggests, where knowledge is imperfect, a space or worksite for the anthropologist opens up. In the case of CKDu, this space or worksite is heavily populated by the work and actions of others. For the anthropologist, this provides an important and productive ethnographic ground. Doctors, scientists, patients, activists, politicians, and journalists are already building the architectures of new diseases, as well as the medicine on which it depends. They are working across distributed and complex communicative fields. By aligning our knowledge-building practices with theirs, we are instructed in the "art of noticing" the processes and connections that matter.

EPILOGUE

In a small village on the shores of Lake Chapala, five-year-old Catalina walks to nursery school. She is showing signs of kidney damage, so says a doctor from a mobile screening unit. As many as 25 percent of her peers are showing similar damage and no one knows why. Is it the food she eats? The lake water she bathes in? The garbage that surrounds her as she bathes? The toxins that her neighbors argue are found in the soil and drinking water? The pesticides her older siblings spray on their family's small patch of land? No one knows. At this point in her young life, no one can be sure whether or not she will develop CKD like her oldest sister, whether or not she will need dialysis or a new kidney. We do know that Catalina is poor and that her family have no entitlements to healthcare, should her kidneys fail. The care she might one day receive, in all likelihood, will establish a trade-off in which the entire wellbeing of her family will be sacrificed for the comparatively short, expensive extension to hers.

In Mexico, for a sizeable population of uninsured kidney patients, regimes of renal care produce hardship rather than health. First-hand acquaintance with those regimes shows that: those with the fewest resources expend all they have to reproduce life at its most fundamental; care for others is individualized and profoundly contingent; a degraded environment, precarious work, and unsafe food threaten the capacity to live well—challenging ontological and bodily security—and become the conditions of emergence for new chronic diseases and harms. In contexts such as these, we encounter the tangled challenges of our time, driving us to ask what can be done to instill a politics of care (Puig de la Bellacasa 2011). This thorny political problem of care acquires renewed urgency when our modes of understanding, persuasion, and intervention no longer seem to work as we once imagined they should; when our human capacities to destroy life seem to have outstripped our capacities to restore it.

It seems appropriate to end this book on that challenge, the challenge of thinking and acting with care, and with more questions than answers. The knotted character of global health concerns—those that reveal the hazardous effects of precarity, environmental harm, and an estrangement from social protections of the sort this book has sought to unpick—compels us to engage in a radical rethink of our orientation to human good and its relation to medical intervention. This is particularly true for a discipline like anthropology, with the human and its ways of life as its central concern.

The need to generate new insights have coalesced in debates about where we find ourselves as a species, in a new era: the Anthropocene. The natural world, we are told, is no longer what conventional science imagined it to be (Haraway et al. 2016). The same goes for our medicine and the diseases it aims to treat. We are also told that the problems we encounter are of our own making; outcomes of our actions—"human species acts." However, this does not help us gain traction on the everyday problem of sickness and the need for care. It is difficult to attribute culpability to what Anna Tsing (in Haraway et al. 2016, 543) refers to as a "concept of undifferentiated mass." The harms that unfold around us cannot easily be distilled to idealizations. If there is a point to the ethnographic exercise, and a place for anthropology as one among other critical interlocutors in getting a measure of and responding to the challenges we face today, it is through our fine-grained "acts of noticing" (Tsing 2015). In other words, it is in our capacity to challenge the uniform and invariable perceptions we have of our world today; to provide release from the generality and sameness that might assume that CKD is CKD the world over and that regimes of renal care come equipped with a uniform set of applications, generating a uniform set of goods. In thinking through the challenges that CKD and renal regimes present for anthropology, it may be that they reveal the need to produce new arguments for much older concerns: poverty, inequality, and the unjust distribution of life chances.

One of the key messages and contributions of this book is to show the importance of bypassing grand categorizations as the starting points for analyses, in order to understand medicine and its effects as the outcomes of the everyday encounters of people. To understand CKD and the regimes of renal care that are bound to it is to see that the intertwining of "cause and care" are products of situated processes: labor and environmental histories; the workings of a political economy; the social and cultural actions of a people at a particular place in time; the product of historical change and struggle. It is only in attending to specificity and detail that we can say something of a more general nature.

And so, as a general reflection on regimes of renal care and their associated technologies, what we can say is that any regime which necessitates radically autonomized individuals and families will not work in any universalized way. Any regime that has the capacity to produce catastrophic poverty and suffering will not produce health overall. Any regime that is predicated on the primacy of hybridized state-medicine-market interests is destined to dis-embed health and welfare from social ties rather than restore them. And any regime that actively ignores the complex conditions of disease emergence, that does not take prevention as it is principal task, will be in no position to respond to growing need. What is more, that CKD disproportionately affects the poor means the trials and labor that accompany attempts to secure care for it, particularly in countries of the so-called globalized south, disproportionately disadvantage them too.

What this book shows is that the entwined social relations of labor, capital, the state, and our lived environment are immediate presences in the lives of people living with CKD and in search of organs for transplant. The Mexican case teaches us that the consolidation of regimes of care is the elaboration of these social relations and that they produce a particular type of politics. Attempts to attend to healthcare without regard for its politics will in the end fail. The Mexican case shows us why.

NOTES

INTRODUCTION

1. Nephrology is a branch of medicine focusing on the kidney.

2. Peritoneal dialysis (PD) is a form of dialysis, where the inside lining of the stomach acts as a natural filter to remove waste products from the blood. Continuous ambulatory peritoneal Dialysis (CAPD) is a common form of PD practiced in Mexico. It is machine-free and done while the patient goes about their everyday activities. It works by way of a catheter (a flexible plastic tube) inserted in the abdomen, which is used to filter fluids into the peritoneal cavity. These fluids remain in the cavity for several hours before being drained out as waste products into an empty bag. This exchange procedure is usually performed four times a day, every day. In hemodialysis, blood is pumped out from the body through a tubing system into an artificial kidney machine, by virtue of a connection called a fistula usually placed in the wrist. It is then returned cleansed to the body via the same connection.

3. Potassium is a mineral present in leafy vegetables and fruits. Healthy kidneys remove excess potassium to help maintain normal levels in the blood. With CKD, this is no longer done efficiently, generating high potassium levels and a condition, called hyperkalemia.

4. Peritonitis is an inflammation of the peritoneum due to infection.

5. The microwave is used to warm the dialysate solution for use in home (peritoneal) dialysis.

6. Muscle cramps are a common complication for patients on hemodialysis.

7. A scapular is a small religious object worn by Catholics, usually made of cloth.

8. Biopsies are part of the diagnostic procedures which help to establish the severity and underlying causes of kidney disease.

9. "Unknown" refers to a new category of CKD that is on the rise and is associated with impoverished social and environmental conditions. It is commonly referred to as chronic kidney disease of unknown origin (CKDu).

10. Social workers in Mexican public health hospitals provide an important conduit between patients and health service access. They are responsible for means-testing patients in order to establish hospital and treatment costs and, as a result, are an important site of negotiation for affordable care. It is difficult to establish either the true costs of CKD or indeed the actual prices that are experienced in common across uninsured Mexican families.

11. Seguro Popular or Popular Health Insurance aims to universalize public health access for the poor. It is described in chapter 2.

12. Antiguo Hospital Civil Viejo "Fray Antonio Alcalde" is part of the Hospitales Civiles Trust together with el Nuevo Hospital Civil de Guadalajara "Dr. Juan I. Menchaca."

13. The inscription and public recognition of these physicians also speak to the dominance and power of the statuses and gender hierarchies that biomedicine often embodies, hierarchies that are as relevant today as they have been throughout the past. As Donna Haraway reminds us in her rich account of Carl Akely, taxonomist and curator of the American Museum of Natural History in New York, public recognition and actual involvement rarely unproblematically align, as behind this "great man" stand a host of unrecognized figures (Haraway 1989).

14. For discussion on the moral and ethical implications of wearing of the "white coat" in hospital ethnography, see Marzano (2007).

15. Biopolitics is a complex and contested concept, emerging with the work of Michel Foucault, to examine the strategies and mechanisms through which life is managed under regimes of authority (Foucault 2003 [1976]). The use and development of the concept has been driven, in large part, by Euro-American approaches, approaches that can lose their relevance when seen in the context of modes of governance in other parts of the world. This is a concern I take up in this book with reference to Mexico.

16. IMSS is the Instituto Mexicano de Seguro Social (the Mexican Institute of Social Security). IMSS provides health insurance for private-sector salaried workers and their families, covering approximately 44 percent of the population. It is Mexico's largest healthcare provider.

17. See reflections on Charles Bowden's (1998) book *Juarez: The Laboratory of Our Future* by Ed Vulliamy writing a critique on capitalism in Mexico in *The Guardian* newspaper on June 20, 2011 (https://www.theguardian.com/commentisfree/2011/jun/20/war-capitalism-mexico-drug-cartels).

CHAPTER 1   STUDYING REGIMES OF RENAL CARE

1. The regulation school or *l'école de la régulation* was established in the early 1970s in order to update Marxian thinking on political economy. It is influenced by the thinking of Karl Polanyi, Charles Bettelheim, and Michel Aglietta, among others.

CHAPTER 2   BIOPOLITICS AND THE ANALYTICS OF A POPULATION ON THE MOVE

1. The United States Renal Data System (USRDS) suggests Mexico (represented by Morelos and Jalisco) is ranked first in incidence and sixth in prevalence of CKD worldwide (with 425 and 1,402 patients per million inhabitants, respectively) (Solis-Vargas, Evangelista-Carrillo, and Puetes-Camacho 2016).

2. PRI or Partido Revolucionario Institucional was established in 1929. Considered the party of the Mexican revolution, it held power for seventy-one years, until defeated in 2000 by PAN, Partido Acción Nacional, under the leadership of Vincente Fox.

3. Incidentally, according to the most recent USRDS report, in Jalisco by 2015, 51 percent of patients were on peritoneal dialysis (PD) and 49 percent on hemodialysis (HD). In some respects a balance between the programs could be said to have been met, but for the wrong reasons. The increase in HD figures resulted from failures in PD, not because HD was explicitly chosen (USRDS 2017). Mendez-Durán et al. (2010) reported a distribution of 66 percent on PD and 34 percent on HD in 127 IMSS hospitals from twenty-one states, but Jalisco and another eleven states were not included.

4. Kidney transplantation for those under the age of eighteen is covered by Seguro Popular; however, immunosuppression is not.

5. Gomez-Dantes et al. (2016) described CKD in Mexico as a serious concern, as the country recorded a 136 percent rise in DALYs (disability-adjusted life-years) since 1990: the world's second highest DALY rate due to CKD.

6. Mexico has among the highest prevalence of obesity and diabetes in the world (International Diabetes Federation, www.idf.org).

7. This includes figures for both IMSS and ISSSTE.

8. These figures add up to more than 100 percent because a person can be enrolled in more than one scheme at a time (INEGI 2016).

9. An article on The Global Nephrology Workforce estimates that there are approximately twelve nephrologists per 1,000 end-stage kidney disease patients or four per million of the population in Mexico (Sharif, Elsayed, and Stack 2016).

10. Many patients talked about coming to similar arrangements with people they knew in order to generate "informal" types of "formal" employment as an attempt to access IMSS insurance.

11. The number of dialysis sessions at IMSS was, at the time, restricted given the large numbers of patients in need of dialysis there.

12. While Seguro Popular did cover this consultation, patients cannot negotiate with them in the same way they do with the social work department within the hospitals. Patients are often left bewildered as to why some services are covered while others are not.

13. Care-giving is a deeply gendered activity in Mexico. Organ donation was often assumed to naturalize the female body as the giver of life and organs, and was thus domesticated, as another form of nurturing or women's work. However, as Crowley-Matoka (2016) points out, this did not translate in actuality. The giving and receiving of organs revealed much more parity, complexity, and contradiction than rendered in discussion or assumed, particularly in a clinical context (see also Solis-Vargas, Evangelista-Carrillo, and Puetes-Camacho 2016).

CHAPTER 3   LABOR

1. My use of the term *autoconstrucción* is borrowed from the popular term for a type of housing often constructed by families as a "self-construction," whereby a family home is built incrementally through a series of extensions over time, to reflect the changing needs of the household. I am using the term in the context of the Mexican welfare state as an analogue to describe the "as and when," politically expedient introduction of various social assistance and entitlement initiatives over the course of a century and a half.

2. For recent discussion on the privatizations of healthcare in Europe, see Dalgren (2014) on the case of Sweden and Pollack (2005) on the UK.

3. Oportunidades is a social assistance program, which works by way of conditional cash transfers. Although it specifically targets children, it has a package of services for older people, which includes health promotion, nutrition, prevention and control of diseases, sexual and reproductive health, and vaccination.

4. Intermittent dialysis, as the name suggests, is a non-continuous form of renal replacement therapy (RRT), provided for brief intervals, often used as bridge to more stable forms of RRT. At Hospital Civil, intermittent peritoneal dialysis was often practiced every two to four weeks, depending on the specific case.

5. There has been much contest over the utility of neoliberalism as a concept across the social sciences. Although it has served to illuminate some key global trends, it is a concept that is insufficiently theorized, too easily deployed, and often obscures and glosses the specificities of its practice across different sites and settings. For an account of recent debates within anthropology, please see coverage of the debate by Eriksen et al. (2015), "The concept of neoliberalism has become an obstacle to the anthropological understanding of the twenty-first century."

6. The foundations of the Mexican welfare state were established in the aftermath of independence from Spain in 1821. Bankrupt, the new state and its institutions struggled to assert an independent political project and to loosen the Catholic Church's grip on public life (Brachet-Márquez 2007). Developing an infrastructure for secular education was to be the main instrument for state building, the principal purpose of welfare in the early stages of Mexico's history as an independent country, and for forging a national identity. However, without the resources to see this project through, the pronouncements by the state would do little to curb the social injustices and divisions that had marked imperialism under Spain. The election of Porfirio Días in 1876 led to an intensification of these divisions, entrenched across his three and a half decades in power (1876–1880; 1884–1911). While this period produced an appearance of relative political stability, that stability rested on state centrism, repression, and the mobilization of allies and elites rather than effective policy making. During it, welfare did not feature prominently as a vehicle for state building, even rhetorically. Those on the margins of Mexican society would be left there, reliant on the church as their benefactor, which unlike the state did commit funds to social support (Valadés 1979). Known as the Porfiriato, this period of Mexican history ended in political and socioeconomic instability, bequeathing Mexican society a poorly integrated infrastructure of services that served to exacerbate social problems, in particular around public health, generating long-lasting divisions between rural and urban Mexico.

7. The infrastructure of the Mexican welfare state has emerged over time as an outcome of a different set of political-economic shifts, the responses to them by successive political administrations, and the manner and degree to which they have sought to hardwire their respective political projects into the Mexican state. This includes, among other things, the way in which the division of responsibilities between and jurisdictions of the social, the market, and the state have been drawn, redrawn, and policed through it over time.

8. It was not until the period after the Mexican Revolution (1910–1920) and the establishment of the 1917 constitution, that a centralized welfare state capable of delivering some services began to exercise control in the field of welfare. This change was initiated by the emergent PRI party (Partido Revolucionario Institucional, the Institutional Revolutionary Party), the political party of the *caudillos* (military strongmen), who won the Mexican revolution and maintained hegemonic power until the 2000s (Gledhill 2015). Nonetheless, progress was slow. While the Mexican constitution of 1917 laid great stress on the labor rights of workers and the importance of social security provision, it was not until the Cardenas government in the 1930s that a formal welfare infrastructure was put in place. It was designed to meet a series of key objectives: to ensure land redistribution in an effort to transform the rural poor or *campesino* into state subjects with land rights; to regulate the relations between capital and labor and to produce a system of social insurance. A limited social insurance system had already been established for civil servants and the armed forces in 1925, soon followed by teachers and workers in the key national industries such as petroleum (Pemex) and the railroads.

9. These repercussions were, of course, not simply a feature of the Mexican economy but felt throughout the global south, as governments shrank their activities, consumer subsidies were cut, and domestic industries lost their protections, often under the oversight of global financial institutions such as the International Monetary Fund (Shefner 2008).

10. The Zapatista uprising was a 1994 rebellion in Mexico, coordinated by the Zapatista Army of National Liberation in response to the signing of NAFTA.

11. Oportunidades was the successor to PROGRESA (Programa de Educación, Salud y Alimenación, the Program for Education, Health and Nutrition)—a program created to address the needs of those living in extreme rural poverty, by providing a mechanism to distribute food, healthcare, and educational scholarships. It was renamed by Vincente Fox after his election in 2000 with an increase in budget of 85 percent in an effort to double its reach.

12. Conditional cash transfers (CCTs) attempt to reduce poverty by making welfare conditional on the receiver meeting a set of established criteria, such as enrolling children in schools, attending healthcare check-ups, and so on. CCTs cover approximately 12 percent of the population in Latin America, with Oportunidades the second largest after Brazil.

13. See article in the *New York Times* addressing Mexico's social contract and its consequences for inequality (Fisher and Taub 2017).

CHAPTER 4   BROKERING HEALTHCARE

1. My thinking here has been shaped by ongoing conversations with Michael Mair over more than a decade. Michael's work offers a situated and political reading of the problem of the state and will be set out in a forthcoming monograph, *The Problem of the State*. I would urge readers to look out for this title once published.

2. Studies of paperwork have gained increasing attention in the anthropological literature. Interest in it covers a rich ground and includes, *inter alia*, attention to its capacity to order administration as well as (re)construct subjects, objects, and social relations (Hull 2012a; Riles 2006); the multiple, messy, and contingent effects of documents (Das and Pool 2004; Navaro-Yashin 2007); the transactions, procedures, and practices that govern the exchange of documents between organizational entities (Appadurai 1986; Strathern 1999); the significance of bureaucratic control through uncertainty or exclusions to the process of documentation (Ticktin 2006) its role in the constitution of disease and treatment (Bowker and Star 1999).

3. I normally accompanied Ana to consultations, squeezing in at one end of the small consultation desk, often taking up the only extra chair. Once again, the consultation rooms are not private spaces—doors are left open with doctors, nurses, and teams of young nutritionists coming and going throughout the day.

4. Tuberculosis is ordinarily associated with the respiratory system but can involve other organ systems. The abdomen is the most common site of extrapulmonary tuberculosis, with peritoneal disease being the most prevalent form within the abdomen.

5. Creatinine is a chemical waste compound that is excreted in the urine. Raised creatinine levels signify impaired kidneys, due to poor clearance functions.

6. Valganciclovir is an antiviral medication used to treat cytomegalovirus (CMV) infection in those with HIV/AIDS or following organ transplant. It is often used long term as it only suppresses rather than cures the infection.

7. Glomerulonephritis or glomerular nephritis is a cluster of kidney diseases often affecting both kidneys, and characterized by inflammation either of the glomeruli or of the small blood vessels in the kidneys.

8. Scott's use of "transcripts"—both hidden and public—relate to established ways of behaving and speaking that reflect social actors in particular social settings, be they dominant or oppressed.

9. For an understanding of moral economy, I draw on Andrew Sayer's use of the term in that it "embodies norms and sentiments regarding the responsibilities and rights of individuals and institutions with respect to others. These norms and sentiments go beyond matters of justice and equality to conceptions of the good" (2000, 79).

10. I borrow from Alex Nading (2017), who draws on the idea of a "crafted bureaucracy" as the written social norms that ensure both the quality of food and the social relations that underpin its production. He suggests this manifests "a shared dignity built into the conduct of government" (2017, 479).

CHAPTER 5   EXCHANGE

1. For further reading on the production and management of debt in Mexican households, Villarreal's (2014) paper on regimes of value and the practical management of debt provides fine-grained insights into the cultural, moral, and economic relations that structure monetary frameworks.

2. These medications include, among other things, drugs for anemia, such as erythropoietin; diuretics for fluid buildup; anti-hypertensive or blood pressure tablets; phosphate binders to control phosphate levels; iron supplements; statins; vitamins; immunosuppressants to prevent organ rejection; steroids; and so on.

3. PiSA has its own pharmacy chain, Farmacias La Paz. Two of these pharmacies were located near the hospital.

4. As Hayden points out, the generic drugs market is the biggest and fastest-growing pharmaceutical market in Latin America.

CHAPTER 6   TRANSPLANT SCANDALS, THE STATE, AND THE "MULTIPLE PROBLEMATICS" OF ACCOUNTABILITY

1. PRD stands for Partido de la Revolución Democrática (Party of the Democratic Revolution).

2. CENATRA (acronym in Spanish for Centro Nacional de Trasplantes) is the National Transplant Council, an agency of the Ministry of Health responsible for national policies and legal frameworks on tissue and organ donation and transplantation and steward of the National Transplant System and the National Transplant Registry.

3. Also the Office of the General Prosecutor of Jalisco, and head of the police state forces and law.

4. See the following media articles: "Emilio González Defiende a Hospitales Civiles" (*Informador* 2008e); "Confirman que Rodríguez Sancho Realizó Cobros Ilegales en Programa de Trasplantes" (*Informador* 2008b).

5. A bad apple defense focuses on the infraction of an individual rather than questioning the role or conduct of the organization.

6. Reported in "Denuncian ante la PGR Presunto Tráfico de Órganos" (*Informador* 2008c).

7. The issue of using fee-paying patients to support those with no resources emerged a number of times in the context of the scandal as a means to justify serving both private and public patients but also as a way to support the return of the surgeon to clinical practice (see "Director de los Civiles Autorizó Trasplantar a Pacientes Particulares," *Informador* 2008d). Given the extent to which patients pay for all aspects of their care—in particular the unpredictable and ancillary costs of renal care—it is unclear what this would look like in practice.

CHAPTER 7   POLITICAL AND CORPORATE ETIOLOGIES

1. Aristolochia is collective term for a large plant genus of over 500 species, commonly known as birthwort or pipevine.

2. These are standard diagnostic tests for identifying the status of kidney functioning.

3. In their analysis of HIV's controversial status as the direct cause of AIDS during the 1990s, Fujimura and Chou show how disputes over the condition's etiology was an outcome of different "styles of scientific practice." Working from a reformulation of Hacking's "styles of scientific reasoning," the authors focused attention on "epidemiological styles of practice," a mosaic or meshing of disciplines, contingent and context dependent, ostensibly a co-production between "field and case study" (Fujimura and Chou 1994, 1023). They suggest that the very organization and nature of epidemiology indicates inter-world activity and joint work, themselves inevitably political.

4. For information on CENCAM, see http://www.regionalnephropathy.org/; for information on La Isla Foundation, see https://laislanetwork.org/.

5. The first media piece raising concerns about CKD around Chapala Lake was published in September 2007 in *Ronda*, titled *Itzicán Poncitlán, Jalisco: Los Olvidados* (The forgotten ones). The article focused on some of the families and patients from one of the lakeside towns.

6. The lake, thought to be one of the dirtiest in Latin America, is an ongoing source of concern for environmental activists, as is the Santiago River, which flows from Chapala Lake to the Pacific Ocean. Over 400 factories have been established along the river and have been dumping waste there for decades. Greenpeace staged a protest along the river in 2012 to mark world water day (see https://phys.org/news/2015-12-pollution-hazardous-foam-mexican-river.htm; Von Bertrab 2003; https://theguadalajarareporter.net/index.php/news/news/guadalajara/30799 -greenpeace-activists-draw-attention-to-polluted-santiago).
7. Chronic conditions have been identified by the WHO as constituting 60 percent of deaths globally today, with 80 percent of these occurring in LMICs (Seeberg and Meinert 2015).
8. For a critical appraisal of the construct of the "epidemiological transition" see (Armstrong 2013)
9. The "nutrition transition" has been coined to mark a shift in dietary consumption and energy expenditure that coincides with economic, demographic, and epidemiological change. Specifically the term is used for the transition of developing countries from traditional diets high in cereal and fiber to more Western-pattern diets high in sugars, fat, and animal-source food (Popkin 1993).
10. Melissa Hogenboom, "Ebola: Is Bushmeat behind the Outbreak?," BBC, October 19, 2014, http://www.bbc.co.uk/news/health-29604204.
11. Bob Wallace is an evolutionary biologist and Roderick Wallace an epidemiologist.

REFERENCES

Adams, Vicanne. 2016. *Metrics: What Counts in Global Health*. Durham, N.C.: Duke University Press.

Agamben, Giorgio. 1998. *Home Sacer: Sovereign Power and Bare Life*. Stanford, Calif.: Stanford University Press.

Agren, David. 2016. "Mexico Cuts Poverty at a Stroke." *The Guardian*, July 18, 2016. https://www .theguardian.com/world/2016/jul/18/mexico-cuts-poverty-national-statistics-changes -earnings-measurements.

Alegre-Díaz, Jesus, William Herrington, Malaguías López-Cervantes, Louisa Gnatiuc, Michael Hill, . . . and Jonathan Emberson. 2017. "Diabetes and Cause-Specific Mortality in Mexico City." *New England Journal of Medicine* 375: 1961–1971.

Appadurai, Arjun. 1986. *The Social Life of Things: Commodities in Cultural Perspective*. Cambridge: Cambridge University Press.

Appadurai, Arjun. 1996. *Modernity at Large: Cultural Dimensions of Globalisation*. Minneapolis: University of Minnesota Press.

Arendt, Hannah. 1998 [1958]. *The Human Condition*. Chicago, Ill.: University of Chicago Press.

Aretxaga, Begona. 1997. *Shattering Silence: Women, Nationalism and Political Subjectivity in Northern Ireland*. Princeton, N.J.: Princeton University Press.

Armstrong, David. 2013. "Chronic Illness: A Revisionist Account." *Sociology of Health and Illness* 36, no. 1: 15–27.

Atilano, Alejandra. 2008a. "Lucran Con Órganos en el Hospital Civil." *Mural*, July 4, 2008, 1.

Atilano, Alejandra. 2008b. "Suspenden Trasplantes." *Mural*, July 6, 2008, 1.

Auyero, Javier. 2000. *Poor People's Politics*. Durham, N.C.: Duke University Press.

Auyero, Javier. 2011. "Patients of the State: An Ethnographic Account of Poor People's Waiting." *Latin American Research Review* 46, no. 1: 5–29.

Avera, Emily. 2009. "Rationalisation and Racialisation in the Rainbow Nation: Inequalities and Identity in the South African Bone Marrow Transplant Network." *Anthropology and Medicine* 16: 179–193.

Ayodele, Olubenga, and Olutayo Alebiosu. 2010. "Burden of Chronic Kidney Disease: An International Perspective." *Advances in Chronic Kidney Disease* 17, no. 3: 215–224.

Baer, Hans, Merill Singer, and Ida Susser. 2003. *Medical Anthropology and the World System*. Santa Barbara, Calif.: Greenwood Publishing Group.

Barba Solano, Carlos. 2007. *¿Reducir la Pobreza o Construir Ciudadan´ia Social para Todos? America Latina: Regimenes de Bienestar en Transicion al Iniciar el Siglo XXI*. Guadalajara: University of Guadalajara Press.

Barba Solano, Carlos, Ivo Anete Brito Leal, Valencia Lomelí Enrique, and Alicia Ziccardi. 2005. "Research Horizon: Poverty in Latin America." In *The Polyscopic Landscape of Poverty Research*. *"State of the Art,"* edited by Else Oyen, 29–60. Bergen, Norway: International Poverty Research, CROP.

Barrientos, Armando, and Leonith Hinojosa-Valencia. 2009. *A Review of Social Protection in Latin America*. Report for Brooks World Poverty Institute, University of Manchester, and the Centre for Social Protection.

Bello, Aminu, David Johnson, John Feehally, David Harris, Kailash Jindal, . . . and Adera Levin. 2017. "Global Kidney Health Atlas (GKHA): Design and Methods." *Kidney International Supplements* 7, no. 2: 145–153.

Biehl, João, and Adriana Petryna. 2013. *When People Come First: Critical Studies in Global Health.* Princeton, N.J.: Princeton University Press.

Bijker, Wiebe. 2007. "Dikes and Dams, Thick with Politics." *Isis* 98, no. 1: 109–123.

Birch, Kean, and David Tyfield. 2012. "Theorizing the Bioeconomy: Biovalue, Biocapital, Bio-economics or . . . What?" *Science, Technology and Human Values* 38, no. 3: 299–327.

Blane, David. 1987. "The Value of Labour-Power and Health." In *Sociological Theory and Medical Sociology*, edited by Graham Scambler, 8–36. London: Tavistock.

Bloor, David. 1991. *Knowledge and Social Imagery.* Chicago, Ill.: University of Chicago Press.

Boltvinik, Julio. 2003. "Welfare, Inequality and Poverty in Mexico, 1979–2000." In *Confronting Development*, edited by Kevin Middlebrook and Eduardo Zepeda, 385–446. Palo Alto, Calif.: Stanford University Press.

Bornstein, Erica. 2009. "The Impulse of Philanthropy." *Cultural Anthropology* 24, no. 4: 622–651.

Bourdieu, Pierre. 1984. *Distinction: A Social Critique of the Judgment of Taste.* Cambridge, Mass.: Harvard University Press.

Bowden, Charles. 1998. *Juarez: The Laboratory of our Future.* New York: Aperture Press.

Bowker, Geoffrey, and Star Susan Leigh. 1999. *Sorting Things Out: Classification and Its Consequences.* Cambridge, Mass.: MIT Press.

Boyer, Robert. 1990. *The Regulation School: A Critical Introduction.* New York, N.Y.: Columbia University Press.

Brachet-Márquez, Viviane. 2007. *Salud Pública y Regímenes de Pensiones en la era Neoliberal.* México: El Colegio de México.

Briggs, Charles, and Clara Mantini-Briggs. 2016. *Tell Me Why My Children Died: Rabies, Indigenous Knowledge and Communicative Justice.* Durham, N.C.: Duke University Press.

Burawoy, Michael. 2000. "A Sociology for the Second Great Transformation?" *Annual Review of Sociology* 26: 693–699.

Callon, Michel. 1986. "Elements of a Sociology of Translation: Domestication of the Scallops and the Fishermen of St Brieuc Bay." In *Power, Action and Belief: A New Sociology of Knowledge*, edited by John Law, 196–233. London: Routledge.

Callon, Michel, and Bruno Latour. 1981. "Unscrewing the Big Leviathan; or How Actors Macrostructure Reality, and How Sociologists Help Them to Do So?" In *Advances in Social Theory and Methodology*, edited by Karin Knorr Cetina and Aaron Cicourel, 277–303. London: Routledge and Kegan Paul.

Cantú Calderon, Ricardo, Antonio Gómez López, and Héctor Villarreal Páez. 2016. "The Labor-Market Deterioration and Its Relation with Poverty during the International Crises in Mexico." Realidad, Datos Y Espacio Revista Internacional de Estadística Y Geografía, *INEGI* 7, no. 3: 1–84.

Cantú-Quintanilla, Guillermo, Josefina Alberú, Rafael Reyes-Acevedo, Mara Medeiros, María De La Salud Villa, . . . and Alfonso Reyes-López. 2011. "A Comparative Study of the Traditional Method, and a Point-Score System for Allocation of Deceased-Donor Kidneys: A National Multicenter Study in Mexico." *Transplant Proceedings* 43, no. 9: 3327–3330.

Cárdenas-González, Mariana, Citlalli Osorio-Yáñez, Octavio Gaspar-Ramírez, Mira Pavkovic, Angeles Ochoa-Martinez, . . . and Vishal Vaidya. 2016. "Environmental Exposure to Arsenic and Chromium in Children is Associated with Kidney Injury Molecule-1." *Environmental Research* 150: 653–662.

Cohen, Lawrence. 2002. "The Other Kidney: Biopolitics beyond Recognition." In *Commodifying Bodies*, edited by Nancy Scheper-Hughes and Loic Wacquant, 9–30. London: Sage.

Cohen, Lawrence. 2004. "Operability." In *Anthropology in the Margins of the State*, edited by Veena Das and Deborah Poole, 165–190. Santa Fe, N.M.: School for Advanced Research Press.

Cohen, Lawrence. 2011. "Migrant Supplementarity: Remaking Biological Relatedness in Chinese Military and Indian Five-Star Hospitals." *Body and Society* 17: 31–54.

Contreras, A. G. 2016. "Organ Transplantation in Mexico." *Transplantation* 100, no. 10: 2011–2012.

Copeman, Jacob. 2009. "Gathering Points: Blood Donation and the Scenography of 'National Integration' in India." *Body and Society* 15: 71–99.

Cordera, Rolando, and Carlos Tello. 2015 [1984]. *La Desigualdad en México*. Mexico: Siglo XXI Editores.

Correa-Rotter, Ricardo, Catharina Wesseling, and Richard Johnson. 2014. "CKD of Unknown Origin in Central America: The Case for a Mesoamerican Nephropathy." *American Journal of Kidney Disease* 63, no. 3: 506–520.

Crowley-Matoka, Megan. 2005. "Desperately Seeking 'Normal': The Promise and Perils of Living with Kidney Transplantation." *Social Science and Medicine* 61: 821–831.

Crowley-Matoka, Megan. 2016. *Domesticating Organ Transplant: Familial Sacrifice and National Aspiration in Mexico*. Durham, N.C.: Duke University Press.

Cusumano, Ana Maria, Rosa-Diez Guillermo, and Maria Gonzalez-Bedat. 2016. "Latin American Dialysis and Transplant Registry: Experience and Contributions to End Stage Renal Disease Epidemiology." *World Journal of Nephrology* 6, no. 5: 389–397.

Dalgren, Gören. 2014. "The Privatization of Medical Health Care in Sweden: Why Public Health Services? Experiences from Profit-Driven Healthcare Reforms in Sweden." *International Journal of Health Services* 44, no. 3: 507–524.

D'Andrade, Roy. 1995. "Moral Models in Anthropology." *Current Anthropology* 36, no.3: 399–408.

Das, Veena. 2001. "Stigma, Contagion, Defect: Issues in the Anthropology of Public Health." Paper Presented at Stigma and Global Health Conference, Bethesda, Md. http://www.stigmaconference.nih.gov/FinalDasPaper.htm#_ftn11. Accessed June 5, 2013.

Das, Veena. 2006. *Life and Worlds: Violence and the Descent into the Ordinary*. Berkeley: University of California Press.

Das, Veena, and Deborah Poole. 2004. *Anthropology in the Margins of the State*. Santa Fe, N.M.: School of American Research Press.

de Laet, Marianne, and Annemarie Mol. 2000. "The Zimbabwe Bush Pump: Mechanics of a Fluid Technology." *Social Studies of Science* 30, no. 2: 225–263.

de Silva, Amarasiri, Steven Albert, and JMKB Jayasekara. 2017. "Structural Violence and Chronic Kidney Disease of Unknown Etiology in Sri Lanka." *Social Science and Medicine* 178: 184–195.

DiGirolamo, Ann, and Nelly Salgado de Snyder. 2008. "Women as Primary Caregivers in Mexico: Challenges to Wellbeing." *Salud Pública de México* 50, no. 6: 516–522.

Douglas, Mary. 1990. "Foreword." In M. Mauss, *The Gift: The Form and Reason for Exchange in Archaic Societies*. London: Routledge.

Eibenschutz, Catalina, Silvia Támez, and Illiana Camacho. 2008. "Inequality and Erroneous Social Policy Produce Inequity in Mexico." *Revista de Salud Pública* 10, no. 1: 119–132.

Engels, Friedrich. 1926 [1845]. *The Condition of the Working-Class in England*. London: Allen and Unwin.

Erickson, Susan. 2016. "Money Matters: Ebola Bonds and Other Migrating Models of Humanitarian Finance." In "Reflections on Global Cooperation and Migration," edited by Marcus Böckenförde, Nadja Krupke, and Phillipp Michaelis, special issue, *Global Dialogues* 13.

Eriksen, Thomas H., James Laidlaw, Jonathan Mair, Martin Keir, and Soumhya Venkatesan. 2015. "The Concept of Neoliberalism Has Become an Obstacle to the Anthropological Understanding of the Twenty-First Century." *Journal of the Royal Anthropological Institute* 21, no. 4: 911–923.

Escobar, Arturo, and Sonia Alvarez. 1992. *The Making of Social Movements in Latin America: Identity, Strategy, and Democracy*. Boulder, Colo.: Westview Press.

Esping-Andersen, Gøsta. 1990. *The Three Worlds of Welfare Capitalism*. Cambridge: Polity Press.

Estévez, Ariadna. 2013. "The Politics of Death in Mexico: Dislocating Human Rights and Asylum Law through Hybrid Agents." *Glocalism: Journal of Culture, Politics and Innovation* 1: 1–28.

Farmer, Paul. 2004. "An Anthropology of Structural Violence." *Cultural Anthropology* 45, no. 3: 305–325.

Farmer, Paul. 2014. "Diary." *London Review of Books* 36, no. 20: 38–39.

Fassin, Didier. 2006. "La Biopolitique N'est Pas Une Politique de la Vie." *Sociologie et Societés* 38, no. 2: 32–47.

Ferguson, James. 1994. *The Anti-politics Machine: Development, Depoliticization, and Bureaucratic Power in Lesotho*. Cambridge: Cambridge University Press.

Ferguson, James, and Akhil Gupta. 2002. "Spatializing States: Towards an Ethnography of Neoliberal Governmentality." *American Ethnologist* 29, no. 4: 981–1002.

Filgueira, Fernando, and Carlos Filgueira. 2002. "Models of Welfare and Models of Capitalism: The Limits of Transferability." In *Models of Capitalism: Lessons for Latin America*, edited by Evelyn Huber, 129–158. Philadelphia: Pennsylvania State University Press.

Fisher, Max, and Amanda Taub. 2017. "The Social Contract Is Broken: Inequality Becomes Deadly in Mexico." *New York Times*, September 30, 2017. https://www.nytimes.com/2017/09/30/world/americas/mexico-inequality-violence-security.html/.

Fleck, Ludwik. 1979 [1935]. *Genesis and Development of a Scientific Fact*. Chicago, Ill.: University of Chicago Press.

Foster, John. 2011. "The Ecology of Marxian Political Economy." *Monthly Review* 63, no. 4. https://monthlyreview.org/2011/09/01/the-ecology-of-marxian-political-economy/.

Foucault, Michel. 1978. "Governmentality." *Lecture at the College de France, 1st of February*. In *The Foucault Reader: Studies in Governmentality*, edited by Graham Burchall, Colin Gordon, and Peter Miller, 87–104. Hemel Hempstead: Harvester Wheatsheaf.

Foucault, Michel. 1980. *The History of Sexuality, Volume 1: An Introduction*. New York, N.Y.: Vintage Books.

Foucault, Michel. 2003 [1975–1976]. "Society Must Be Defended." In *Lectures at the Collège de France*, translated by David Macy. New York, N.Y.: Picador Press.

Fox, Renee, and Judith Swazey. 1992. *Spare Parts: Organ Replacement in American Society*. Oxford: Oxford University Press.

Frenk, Julio, Eduardo González-Pier, Octavio Gómez-Dantés, Miguel Lezana, and Felicia Knaul. 2006. "Comprehensive Reform to Improve Health System Performance in Mexico." *Lancet* 368: 1524–1534.

Fujimura, Joan, and Danny Chou. 1994. "Dissent in Science: Styles of Scientific Practice and the Controversy over the Cause of Aids." *Social Science and Medicine* 38, no. 8: 1017–1036.

Gálvez, Alyshia. 2018. *Eating NAFTA: Trade, Food Policies, and the Destruction of Mexico*. Berkeley: University of California Press.

Garcia-Diaz, Rocio, and Sandra Sosa-Rubi. 2011. "Analysis of the Distributional Impact of Out-of-Pocket Health Payments: Evidence from a Public Health Insurance Program for the Poor in Mexico." *Journal of Health Economics* 30, no. 4: 707–718.

Garcia-Garcia, Guillermo, and Jonathan Chavez-Iñignez. 2018. "The Tragedy of Having ESRD in Mexico." *Kidney International Reports* 3, no. 5: 1027–1029.

Garcia-Garcia, Guillermo, and Vivekanand Jha. 2015. "CKD in Disadvantaged Populations." *Canadian Journal of Kidney, Health and Disease* 2, no. 18: 1–5.

Garcia-Garcia, Guillermo, Francisco J. Monteon-Ramos, Héctor Garcia-Bejarano, Benjamin Gómez-Navarro, Imelda Hernandez-Reyes, . . . and Normal Ruíz-Morales. 2005. "Renal Replacement Therapy among Disadvantaged Populations in Mexico: A Report from the Jalisco Dialysis and Transplant Registry." *Kidney International* 68, no. 97: S58–S61.

Garcia-Garcia, Guillermo, Karina Renoirte-Lopez, and Isela Marquez-Magaña. 2010. "Disparities in Renal Care in Jalisco, Mexico." *Seminars in Nephrology* 30: 3–7.

Garcia-Garcia, Guillermo, Ricardo Rubio, Melina Amador, Margarita Ibarra-Hernández, Librado de la Torre-Campos, and Francisco Gonzalo Rodríguez García. 2017. "CKDu in Mexican Children: The Case of Poncitlan, Jalisco, Abstract." *Journal of American Society of Nephrology* 28: 767.

García-Trabanino, Ramón, Manuel Cerdas, Magdalena Madero, Kristina Jakobsson, Joaquín Barnoya, and Ricardo Correa-Rotter. 2017. "Nefropatía Mesoamericana: Revisión Breve Basada en el Segundo Taller del Consorcio para el Studio de la Epidemia de Nefropatía en Centroamérica y México (CENCAM)." *Nefrología Latinoamericana* 14, no. 1: 39–45.

Garfinkel, Harold. 1984 [1967]. *Studies in Ethnomethodology*. Cambridge: Polity Press.

Gaspar De Alba, Alicia. 2010. *Making a Killing: Femicide, Free Trade and La Frontera*. Austin: University of Texas Press.

Gledhill, John. 2015. *The New War on the Poor: The Production of Insecurity in Latin America*. Chicago, Ill.: Zed Books.

Goffman, Erving. 1961. *Essays on the Social Situation of Mental Patients and Other Inmates*. New York, N.Y.: Anchor Books.

Gomez-Dantes, Héctor, Nancy Fullman, Héctor Lamadrid-Figueroa, Lucero Cahuana-Hurtado, Leticia Darney, . . . and Ricardo Correa-Rotter. 2016. "Dissonant Health Transition in the States of Mexico, 1990–2013: A Systematic Analysis for the Global Burden of Disease Study 2013." *The Lancet* 388, no. 10058: 2386–2402.

Goodman, Nelson. 1978. *Ways of Worldmaking*. Indianapolis, Ind.: Hackett.

Goody, Jack. 1968. *Literacy in Traditional Societies*. Cambridge: Cambridge University Press.

Gordillo, Gastón. 2014. *Rubble: The Afterlife of Destruction*. Durham, N.C.: Duke University Press.

Gordon, Elisa. 2002. "What 'Race' Cannot Tell Us about Access to Kidney Transplantation." *Cambridge Quarterly of Healthcare Ethics* 11: 134–141.

Gracida-Juárez, Carmen, Ramón Espinoza-Pérez, Jorge Cancin-López, Araceli Ibarra-Villanueva, Urbano Cedillo-López, . . . and Julio César Martínez Álvarez. 2011. "Kidney Transplant Experience at the Specialty Hospital Bernardo Sepulveda National Medical Center Century XXI, Mexican Institute of Social Security." *Revista de Investigación Clínica* 63, no. 1: 19–24.

Grollman, Arthur, John Scarborough, and Bojan Jelaković. 2009. "Aristolochic Acid Nephropathy: An Environmental and Iatrogenic Disease." In *Advances in Molecular Toxicology*, vol. 3, edited by James Fishbein and Jacqueline Heilman, 211–222. Amsterdam: Elsevier.

Gupta, Akhil. 1995. "Blurred Boundaries: The Discourse of Corruption, the Culture of Politics and the Imagined State." *American Ethnologist* 22, no. 2: 375–402.

Gupta, Akhil. 2012. *Red Tape: Bureaucracy, Structural Violence and Poverty in India*. Durham N.C.: Duke University Press.

Gutierrez-Padilla, Jose, Martha Mendoza-Garcia, Salvador Plascencia-Perez, Karina Renoirte-Lopez, Guillermo Garcia-Garcia, . . . and Marcello Tonelli. 2010. "Screening for CKD and Cardiovascular Disease Risk Factors Using Mobile Clinics in Jalisco, Mexico." *American Journal of Kidney Disease* 55, no. 3: 474–484.

Habermas, Jurgen. 1984. *The Theory of Communicative Action*, vol. 1, *Reason and Rationalisation of Society*. Boston, Mass.: Beacon Press.

Hacking, Ian. 1995. *Rewriting the Soul: Multiple Personality and the Science of Memory*. Princeton, N.J.: Princeton University Press.

Hacking, Ian. 2006. "Making Up People." *London Review of Books* 28, no. 16:18–21.

Haller, Dieter, and Chris Shore. 2005. *Corruption: Anthropological Perspectives*. London: Pluto Press.

Hamdy, Sherine. 2010. "The Organ Transplant Debate in Egypt: A Social Anthropological Analysis." *Droit et Cultures* 59: 357–365.

Hamdy, Sherine. 2012. *Our Bodies Belong to God: Organ Transplants, Islam, and the Struggle for Human Dignity in Egypt*. Berkeley: University of California Press.

Hanson, John. 2015. "The Anthropology of Giving: Toward a Cultural Logic of Charity." *Journal of Cultural Economy* 8, no. 4: 501–520.

Haraway, Donna. 1989. *Primate Visions: Gender, Race and Nature in the Posthuman Age*. New York, N.Y.: Routledge.

Haraway, Donna. 1991. *Simians, Cyborgs and Women: The Reinvention of Nature*. New York, N.Y.: Routledge.

Haraway, Donna, Noboru Ishikawa, Scott F. Gilbert, Kenneth Olwig, Anna L. Tsing, and Nils Bubandt. 2016. "Anthropologists Are Talking—about the Anthropocene." *Ethnos* 81, no. 3: 535–564.

Hardt, Michael, and Antonio Negri. 2000. *Empire*. Boston, Mass.: Harvard University Press.

Hastrup, Kirsten. 2016. "A History of Climate Change: Inughuit Responses to Changing Ice Conditions in North-West Greenland." *Climatic Change* 151, no. 1: 67–78.

Hayden, Cori. 2007a. "A Generic Solution? Pharmaceuticals and the Politics of the Similar in Mexico." *Current Anthropology* 48, no. 4: 475–495.

Hayden, Cori. 2007b. "Taking as Giving: Bioscience, Exchange, and the Politics of Benefit-Sharing." *Social Studies of Science* 37, no. 5: 729–758.

Healy, Kieran. 2004. "Altruism as an Organizational Problem: The Case of Organ Procurement." *American Sociological Review* 69: 387–404.

Helmreich, Stefan. 2007. "Blue-green Capital, Biotechnological Circulation and an Oceanic Imaginary: A Critique of Biopolitical Economy." *BioSocieties* 2, no. 3: 287–302.

Herzfeld, Michael. 1992. *The Social Production of Indifference: Exploring the Symbolic Roots of Western Bureaucracy*. Oxford: Berg.

Hogel, Linda. 1999. *Recovering the Nation's Body: Cultural Memory, Medicine and the Politics of Redemption*. New Brunswick, N.J.: Rutgers University Press.

Holmes, Douglas. 2013. *Economy of Words: Communicative Imperatives in Central Banks*. Chicago, Ill.: University of Chicago Press.

Holmes, Douglas, and George Marcus. 2008. "Cultures of Expertise and the Management of Globalisation: Towards a Re-functioning of Ethnography." In *Global Assemblages: Technology, Politics and Ethics as Anthropological Problems*, edited by Aihwa Ong and Stephen Collier, 235–252. Oxford: Blackwell.

Hull, Matthew. 2012a. "Documents and Bureaucracy." *Annual Review of Anthropology* 41, no. 1: 251–267.

Hull, Matthew. 2012b. *Government of Paper: The Materiality of Bureaucracy in Urban Pakistan*. Berkeley: University of California Press.

Ikels, Charlotte. 2013. "The Anthropology of Organ Transplantation." *Annual Review of Transplantation* 42: 89–102.

INEGI (Instituto Nacional de Estadística, Geografía e Informática). 2011. *Censo de Población y Vivienda 2010*. https://www.inegi.org.mx/programas/ccpv/2010/default.html.

INEGI. 2016. *Encuesta Intercensal 2015*. https://www.inegi.org.mx/programas/intercensal/2015/default.html.

Informador. 2008a. "Arraigan Luis Carlos Rodriquez Sancho por Presunto Tráfico de Orgános." *Informador*, July 10, 2008. www.informador.mx/Jalisco/Arraigan-a-Luis-Carlos-Rodriguez-Sancho-por-presunto-trafico-de-organos-20080710-0178.html.

Informador. 2008b. "Confirman que Rodríguez Sancho Realizó Cobros Ilegales en Programa de Trasplantes." *Informador*, July 11, 2008.

Informador. 2008c. "Denuncian ante la PGR Presunto Tráfico de Órganos." *Informador*, August 5, 2008. https://www.informador.mx/Jalisco/Denuncian-ante-la-PGR-presunto-trafico-de-organos-20080805-0084.html.

Informador. 2008d. "Director de los Civiles Autorizo Trasplantar a Pacientes Particulares." *Informador*, September 29, 2008. https://www.informador.mx/Jalisco/Director-de-los-Civiles-autorizo-trasplantar-a-pacientes-particulares-20080929-0274.html.

Informador. 2008e. "Emilio-Gonzalez Defiende a Hospitales Civiles." *Informador*, July 10, 2008. https://www.informador.mx/Jalisco/Emilio-Gonzalez-defiende-a-hospitales-civiles-20080710-0030.html.

Informador. 2008f. "UdeG Aguarda Investigaciones en Hospital Civil." *Informador*, July 10, 2008. https://www.informador.mx/Jalisco/UdeG-aguarda-investigaciones-en-Hospital-Civil-20080710-0022.html.

Ingold, Tim. 2000. *The Perception of the Environment: Essays on Livelihood, Dwelling and Skill*. London: Routledge.

Jackson, Michael. 2005. *Existential Anthropology: Events, Exigencies and Effects*. New York, N.Y.: Berghahn Books.

Jones, Paul, and Michael Mair. 2016. "Genealogy, Parasitism and Moral Economy: The Case of UK Supermarket Growth." In *Neoliberalism and the Moral Economy of Fraud*, edited by David Whyte and Jorg Wiegratz, 86–98. London: Routledge.

Kantola, Anu, and Juho Vesa. 2013. "Mediated Scandals as Social Dramas: Transforming the Moral Order in Finland." *Acta Sociologica* 56 , no. 4: 295–308.

Kierans, Ciara. 2005. "Narrating Kidney Disease: The Significance of Sensation and Time in the Emplotment of Patient Experience." *Culture, Medicine and Psychiatry* 29: 341–359.

Kierans, Ciara. 2011. "Anthropology, Organ Transplantation and the Immune System: Resituating Commodity and Gift Exchange." *Social Science and Medicine* 73: 1469–1476.

Kierans, Ciara. 2014. "Organ Transplantation in Mexico: The Anthropology of an Ambivalent Technology." In *Körperökonomien: Der Körper im Zeitalter seiner Handelbarkeit*, edited by Lea Schumacher and Oliver Decker, 123–142. Berlin: Psychosozial-Verlag.

Kierans, Ciara. 2015. "Biopolitics and Capital: Poverty, Mobility and the Body in Transplantation in Mexico." *Body and Society* 21, no. 3: 42–65.

Kierans, Ciara, and Jessie Cooper. 2011. "Organ Donation, Genetics, Race and Culture: The Making of a Medical Problem." *Anthropology Today* 27, no. 6: 21–25.

Knaul, Felicia, Eduardo González-Pier, Octavio Gómez-Dantes, David García-Junco, Hector Arreola-Ornelas, . . . and Julio Frenk. 2012. "The Quest for Universal Health Coverage: Achieving Social Protection for All in Mexico." *The Lancet* 380, no. 9849: 1259–1279.

Koenig, Barbara. 2003. "Dead Donors and the 'Shortage' of Human Organs: Are We Missing the Point?" *American Journal of Bioethics* 3, no. 1: 26–27.

Korpi, Walter. 2000. "Faces of Inequality: Gender, Class and Patterns of Inequalities in Different Types of Welfare States." *Social Politics: International Studies in Gender State and Society* 7, no. 2: 127–191.

La Isla Foundation. 2015. *The Epidemic*. laislafoundation.org/epidemic/. Accessed May 19, 2017.

Lange Neuen, Brendon, Steven Chadban, Alesandro Demaio, David Johnson, and Vlado Pekovic. 2017. "Chronic Kidney Disease and the Global NCDs Agenda." *BMJ Global Health* 2, no. 2: e000380.

Latour, Bruno. 1987. *Science in Action: How to Follow Scientists and Engineers through Society.* Milton Keynes: Open University Press.

Latour, Bruno. 1999. "Give Me a Laboratory and I Will Raise the World." In *The Science Studies Reader,* edited by Mario Biagioli, 258–275. New York, N.Y.: Routledge.

Latour, Bruno. 2004. "Why Has Critique Run out of Steam? From Matters of Fact to Matters of Concern." *Critical Inquiry* 30, no. 2: 225–248.

Latour, Bruno. 2005. *Reassembling the Social: An Introduction to Actor-Network Theory.* Oxford: Oxford University Press.

Latour, Bruno, and Peter Weibel. 2005. *Making Things Public: Atmospheres of Democracy.* Cambridge, Mass.: MIT Press.

Latour, Bruno, and Steve Woolgar. 1979. *Laboratory Life: The Construction of Scientific Facts.* Princeton, N.J.: Princeton University Press.

Laurell, Asa Christina. 2011. "Los Seguros de Salud Mexicanos: Cobertura Universal Incierta." *Ciência y Saúde Colectiva* 16, no. 6: 2796–2806.

Laurell, Asa Christina. 2015. "The Mexican Popular Health Insurance: Myths and Realities." *International Journal of Health Services* 45, no. 1: 105–125.

Lemke, Thomas. 2011. *Bio-Politics: An Advanced Introduction.* New York, N.Y.: New York University Press.

Levin, Adeera, Marcelo Tonelli, Joseph Bonventure, Joseph Cresh, Jo-Ann Donner, . . . and Kai Uwe Eckardt. 2017. "Global Kidney Health 2017 and Beyond: A Roadmap for Closing Gaps in Care, Research and Policy." *The Lancet* 390, no. 10105: 1888–1917.

Lewis, Oscar. 1961. *The Children of Sanchez.* New York, N.Y.: Random House.

Livingstone, Julia. 2012. *Improving Medicine: An African Oncology Ward in an Emerging Cancer Epidemic.* Durham, N.C.: Duke University Press.

Lock, Margaret. 1995. "Transcending Mortality: Organ Transplants and the Practice of Contradictions." *Medical Anthropology Quarterly* 9, no. 3: 390–393.

Lock, Margaret. 2001. *Twice Dead: Organ Transplants and the Reinvention of Death.* Berkeley: University of California Press.

Lundin, Susanne. 2010. "Organ Economy: Organ Trafficking in Moldova and Israel." *Public Understanding of Science* 1: 1–16.

Lynch, Michael. 1993. *Scientific Practice and Ordinary Action: Ethnomethodology and Social Studies of Science.* New York, N.Y.: Cambridge University Press.

Lynch, Michael. 2008. "Ontography: Investigating the Production of Things, Deflating Ontology." Unpublished, prepared for Oxford Ontologies Workshop, Saïd Business School, Oxford University, June 25, 2008.

Manderson, Lenore. 2011. *Surface Tensions: Surgery, Bodily Boundaries and the Social Self.* Walnut Creek, Calif.: Left Coast Press.

Martín-Cleary, Catalina, and Alberto Ortiz. 2014. "CKD Hotspots around the World: Where, Why and What the Lessons Are. A CKJ Review Series." *Clinical Kidney Journal* 7: 519–523.

Martínez Franzoni, Juliana. 2008. "Welfare Regimes in Latin America: Capturing Constellations of Markets, Families and Policies." *Latin American Politics and Society* 50, no. 2: 67–100.

Marx, Karl. 1970 [1844]. *Economic and Philosophical Manuscripts of 1844.* London: Lawrence and Wishart.

Marx, Karl. 1974 [1867]. *Capital.* 3 vols. London: Lawrence and Wishart.

Marx, Karl. 1998 [1932]. *The German Ideology. Literary Theory: An Anthology.* 2nd ed. Oxford: Blackwell.

Marzano, Marco. 2007. "Informed Consent, Deception, and Research Freedom in Qualitative Research: A Cross-Cultural Comparison." *Qualitative Inquiry* 13, no. 3: 417–436.

Massey, Doreen. 2005. *For Space.* London: Sage.

Mauss, Marcel. 1990 [1950]. *The Gift: The Form and Reason for Exchange in Archaic Societies.* New York, N.Y.: W. W. Norton.

Méndez-Durán, Antonio, Francisco J. Méndez-Bueno, Teresa Tapia-Yáñez, Angélica Muñoz-Montes, and Leticia Aguilar-Sánchez. 2010. "Epidemiología de la insuficiencia renal crónica en México." *Diálisis y Trasplante* 31, no. 1: 7–11.

Mesa-Lago, Carmelo. 1978. *Social Security in Latin America: Pressure Groups, Stratification, and Inequity.* Pittsburgh, Pa.: University of Pittsburgh Press.

Miller, Peter, and Nicholas Rose. 2008. *Governing the Present: Administering Economic, Social and Personal Life.* Cambridge: Polity Press.

Moghadam, Valentine. 2005. "The 'Feminization of Poverty' and Women's Human Rights." *SHS Papers in Women's Studies/Gender Research, Unesco,* no. 2: 1–39.

Mol, Annemarie. 2002. *The Body Multiple: Ontology in Medical Practice.* Durham, N.C.: Duke University Press.

Mol, Annemarie. 2008. *The Logic of Care: Health and the Problem of Patient Choice.* London: Routledge.

Montoya, Michael. 2011. *Making the Mexican Diabetic: Race, Science and the Genetics of Inequality.* Berkeley: University of California Press.

Murai, Tomoko. 2004. "The Foundation of the Mexican Welfare State and Social Security Reform in the 1990s." *The Developing Economies* 42, no. 2: 262–287.

Murray, Christopher, Allan Lopez, Mohsen Naghavi, and Haidong Wang. 2016. "Global, Regional and National Life Expectancy, All-Cause Mortality, and Cause-Specific Mortality for 249 Causes of Death, 1980–2015: A Systematic Analysis for the Global Burden of Disease Study 2015." *The Lancet* 388, no. 10053: 1459–1544.

Nading, Alex. 2017. "Orientation and Crafted Bureaucracy: Finding Dignity in Nicaraguan Food Safety." *American Anthropologist* 119, no. 3: 478–490.

Nading, Alex, and Lucy Lowe. 2018. "Social Justice as Epidemic Control: Two Latin American Case Studies." *Medical Anthropology* 37, no. 6: 458–471.

National Kidney Foundation. 2012. "Factsheets." http://www.organdonation.nhs.uk/newsroom /fact_sheets/cost_effectiveness_of_transplantation.asp.

Navaro-Yashin, Yael. 2002. *Faces of the State: Secularism and Public Life in Turkey.* Princeton, N.J.: Princeton University Press.

Navaro-Yashin, Yael. 2007. "Make-believe Papers, Legal Forms and the Counterfeit: Affective Interactions between Documents and People in Britain and Cyprus." *Anthropology Theory* 7, no. 1: 79–98.

Nguyen, Vinh-Kim, and Karine Peschard. 2003. "Anthropology, Inequality and Disease: A Review." *Annual Review of Anthropology* 32: 447–474.

Nielsen, Kristian, and Mads P. Sørensen. 2015. "How to Take Non-knowledge Seriously, or 'The Unexpected Virtue of Ignorance.'" *Public Understanding of Science* 26, no. 3: 385–392.

Novas, Carlos. 2006. "The Political Economy of Hope: Patients' Organizations, Science and Biovalue." *BioSocieties* 1: 289–305.

OECD. 2017. *How's Life in Mexico?* https://www.oecd.org/statistics/Better-Life-Initiative -country-note-Mexico.pdf.

Ong, Aihwa. 1999. *Flexible Citizenship: The Cultural Logics of Transnationality.* Durham, N.C.: Duke University Press.

Oniscu, Gabriel, and John Forsythe. 2009. "An Overview of Transplantation in Culturally Diverse Regions." *Annals Academy of Medicine Singapore* 38, no. 4: 365–369.

Padilla-Altamira, Cesar. 2017. *Healthcare at the Margins: An Ethnography of Chronic Kidney Disease and Peritoneal Dialysis in Mexico.* PhD thesis, University of Liverpool.

Pan American Health Organization. 2014. "PAHO Resolution CD52.R1.: Chronic Kidney Disease in Agricultural Communities in Central America." http://www.paho.org/hq/index.php ?option=com_content&view=article&id=8833&Itemid=40033&lang=en.

Paniagua, Ramón, Alfonso Ramos, Rosaura Fabian, Jesús Lagunas, and Dante Amato. 2007. "Chronic Kidney Disease and Dialysis in Mexico." *Peritoneal Dialysis International* 27, no. 4: 405–409.

Parsons, Talcott. 1940. "An Analytical Approach to the Theory of Social Stratification." *American Journal of Sociology* 45, no. 6: 841–862.

Parsons, Talcott. 1951. *The Social System.* Glencoe Ill.: The Free Press.

Pavlovic, Nicola. 2013. "Balkan Endemic Nephropathy: Current Status and Future Perspectives." *Clinical Kidney Journal* 6, no. 3: 257–265.

Pedersen, Susan. 2018 "One-Man Ministry." *London Review of Books* 40, no. 3: 3–6.

Petryna, Adrianna. 2002. *Life Exposed: Biological Citizens after Chernobyl.* Princeton, N.J.: Princeton University Press.

Polayni, Karl. 2001 [1944]. *The Great Transformation: The Political and Economic Origins of Our Time.* Boston, Mass.: Beacon Press.

Pollack, Alison. 2005. *NHS Plc: The Privatization of our Health Care.* London: Verso Books.

Popkin, Barry. 1993. "Nutritional Patterns and Transitions." *Population and Development Review* 19, no. 1: 138–157.

Portes, Alejandro, and Kelly Hoffman. 2003. "Latin American Class Structures: Their Composition and Change during the Neoliberal Era." *Latin American Research Review* 38, no. 1: 41–82.

Puig de la Bellacasa. 2011. "Matters of Care in Technoscience: Assembling Neglected Things." *Social Studies of Science* 41, no. 1: 85–106.

Rabinow, Paul, and Nicolas Rose. 2006. "Biopower Today." *Biosocieties* 1, no. 2:195–217.

Race, Kane. 2012. "Frequent Sipping: Bottled Water, the Will to Health and the Subject of Hydration." *Body and Society* 18, nos. 3–4: 72–98.

Ramirez-Rubio, Orina, Michael McClean, Juan Jose Amador, and Daniel Brooks. 2013. "An Epidemic of Chronic Kidney Disease in Central America: An Overview." *Postgraduate Medical Journal* 89, no. 1049: 123–125.

Rappert, Brian. 2012. *How to Look Good in War.* London: Pluto Press.

Resa, Gloria M. 2008. "Desintrés de las Autoridades." *Processo,* July 20, 2008, 193.

Riles, Annelise. 2006. *Documents: Artifacts of Modern Knowledge.* Ann Arbor: University of Michigan Press.

Rose, Nicholas. 2007. *The Politics of Life Itself: Biomedicine, Power, and Subjectivity in the Twenty-First Century.* Princeton, N.J.: Princeton University Press.

Rose, Nicholas, and Peter Miller. 2010. "Political Power beyond the State: Problematics of Government." *British Journal of Sociology* 61, no. 1: 271–303.

Rose, Nicholas, and Carlos Novas. 2005. "Biological Citizenship." In *Global Assemblages: Technology, Politics and Ethics as Anthropological Problems,* edited by Aiwha Ong and Stephen Collier, 439–463. Malden, Mass.: Blackwell.

Ruppert, Evelyn. 2012. "The Governmental Topologies of Database Devices." *Theory, Culture and Society* 29, nos. 4–5: 1–21.

Ryle, Gilbert. 1949. *The Concept of Mind.* Chicago, Ill.: University of Chicago Press.

Sahlins, Marshal. 1963. "Poor Man, Rich Man, Big Man, Chief: Political Types in Melanesia and Polynesia." *Comparative Studies in Society and History* 5, no. 3: 285–303.

Sanal, Aslihan. 2011. *New Organs within Us: Transplants and the Moral Economy.* Durham, N.C.: Duke University Press.

Sayer, Andrew. 2000. "Moral Economy and Political Economy." *Studies in Political Economy* 61: 79–103.

Scheper-Hughes, Nancy. 2000. "The Global Traffic in Human Organs." *Current Anthropology* 41, no. 2: 191–224.

Scheper-Hughes, Nancy. 2008. "The Last Commodity." *Dissenting Knowledges* pamphlet series, no. 6: 1–55.

Schneider, Ben, and David Soskice. 2009. "Inequality in Developed Countries and Latin America: Coordinated, Liberal and Hierarchical Systems." *Economy and Society* 38, no. 1: 17–52.

Scott, James. 1972. *Comparative Political Corruption.* Englewood Cliffs, N.J.: Prentice Hall.

Scott, James. 1990. *Domination and the Arts of Resistance: Hidden Transcripts.* New Haven, Conn.: Yale University Press.

Scott, James. 1998. *Seeing Like a State: How Certain Schemes to Improve the Human Condition Have Failed.* New Haven, Conn.: Yale University Press.

Seeberg, Jens, and Lotte Meinert. 2015. "Can Epidemics Be Noncommunicable? Reflections on the Spread of 'Noncommunicable Diseases.'" *Medicine Anthropology Theory* 2, no. 2: 54–71.

Shapin, Steven, and Simon Schaffer. 1985. *Leviathan and the Airpump: Hobbes, Boyle and the Experimental Life.* Princeton, N.J.: Princeton University Press.

Sharif, Muhammad, Mohamed E. Elsayed, and Austin G. Stack. 2016. "The Global Nephrology Workforce: Emerging Threats and Potential Solutions." *Clinical Kidney Journal* 9, no. 1: 11–22.

Sharma, Aradhana, and Akhil Gupta. 2006. *The Anthropology of the State: A Reader.* Malden, Mass.: Blackwell.

Sharp, Lesley. 2000. "The Commodification of the Body and Its Parts." *Annual Review of Anthropology* 29: 287–328.

Sharp, Lesley. 2006. *Strange Harvest: Organ Transplants, Denatured Bodies, and the Transformed Self.* Berkeley: University of California Press.

Sharp, Lesley. 2013. *The Transplant Imaginary: Mechanical Hearts, Animal Parts, and Moral Thinking in Highly Experimental Science.* Berkeley: University of California Press.

Shefner, Jon. 2008. *The Illusion of Civil Society: Democratization and Community Mobilization in Low-Income Mexico.* University Park: Pennsylvania State University Press.

Shimazono, Yosuke. 2007. "The State of the International Organ Trade: A Provisional Picture based on Integration of Available Information." *Bulletin of the World Health Organization* 85: 955–962.

Shimazono, Yosuke. 2008. "Repaying and Cherishing the Gift of Life: Gift Exchange and Living Related Kidney Transplantation in the Philippines." *Anthropology in Action* 15, no. 3: 34–46.

Solis-Vargas, E., L. Evangelista-Carrillo, and A. Puetes-Camacho. 2016. "Epidemiological Characteristics of the Largest Kidney Transplant Program in Mexico: Western National Medical Center, Mexican Institute of Social Security." *Transplantation Proceedings* 48: 1999–2005.

Spivak, Gayatri. 2003. *Death of a Discipline.* New York, N.Y.: Columbia University Press.

Stanifer, John, Anthony Muiru, Tazeen Jafars, and Uptal Patel. 2016. "Chronic Kidney Disease in Low- and Middle-Income Countries." *Nephrology Dialysis Transplantation* 31: 868–874.

Strathern, Andrew. 1974. *Ongka's Big Moka: The Kawelka of Papua New Guinea.* Directed by Charlie Nairn. Great Britain: Disappearing World Series.

Strathern, Marilyn. 1999. *Property, Substance, Effect: Anthropological Essays on Persons and Things.* London: Athlone.

Strathern, Marilyn. 2009. "Afterword." *Body and Society* 15, no. 2: 217–222.

Sunder, Rajan Kaushik. 2006. *Biocapital.* Durham, N.C.: Duke University Press.

Sunder, Rajan Kaushik. 2012. *Lively Capital: Biotechnologies, Ethics and Governance in Global Markets.* Durham, N.C.: Duke University Press.

Támez, Silvia, and Catalina Eibenschutz. 2008. "Popular Health Insurance: Key Piece of Inequity in Health in Mexico." *Revista de Salud Pública* 10: 133–145.

Taussig, Michael. 1980. *The Devil and Commodity Fetishism in South America.* Chapel Hill: University of North Carolina Press.

Ticktin, Miriam. 2006. "Where Ethics and Politics Meet: The Violence of Humanitarianism in France." *American Ethnologist* 33, no. 1: 33–49.

Torsello, Davide. 2010. "Corruption and the Economic Crisis: Empirical Indications from Eastern Europe." *Slovak Foreign Policy Affairs* 19, no. 2: 65–75.

Trabanino, Ramón, Raul Aguilar, Carlos Silva, Manuel Mercado, and Ricardo Merino. 2002. "End-Stage Renal Disease among Patients in a Referral Hospital in El Salvador." *Revista Panamericana de Salud Pública* 12, no. 3: 202–206.

Treviño-Becerra, Alejandro. 2007. "The Mexican Peritoneal Dialysis Model: A Personal Reflection." *Artificial Organs* 31, no. 4: 249–252.

Trnka, Susanna, and Catherine Trundle. 2014. "Competing Responsibilities: Moving beyond Neoliberal Responsibilization." *Anthropological Forum* 24, no. 2: 136–153.

Tsing, Anna. 2005. *Friction: An Ethnography of Global Connection.* Princeton, N.J.: Princeton University Press.

Tsing, Anna. 2009. "Supply Chains and the Human Condition." *Journal of Economics, Culture & Society* 21, no. 2: 148–176.

Tsing, Anna. 2013. "Sorting Out Commodities: How Capitalist Value Is Made through Gifts." *HAU: Journal of Ethnographic Theory* 3, no. 1: 21–43.

Tsing, Anna. 2015. *The Mushroom at the End of the World: On the Possibility of Life in Capitalist Ruins.* Princeton, N.J.: Princeton University Press.

Tutton, Richard. 2002. "Gift Relationship in Genetics Research." *Science as Culture* 11, no. 4: 523–542.

U.S. Department of Health and Human Services. 2013. *The Living Donation Process.* http://organdonor.gov/about/livedonation.html.

USRDS. 2017. *2017 USRDS Annual Data Report: Epidemiology of Kidney Disease in the United States. Volume 2: End-Stage Renal Disease in the United States.* Bethesda, Md.: National Institutes of Health, National Institute of Diabetes and Digestive and Kidney Diseases.

Valadés, José C. 1979. *Historia General de la Revolución Mexicana.* Vol. 2. 2nd ed. México: Editorial del Valle de México.

Valencia Lomelí, Enrique. 2008. "Conditional Cash Transfers as Social Policy in Latin America: An Assessment of Their Contributions and Limitations." *Annual Review of Sociology* 34: 475–499.

Varul, Matthias. 2010. "Talcott Parsons, the Sick Role and Chronic Illness." *Body and Society* 16, no. 2: 72–94.

Verduzco Igartúa, Gustavo. 2003. *Organizaciones no Lucrativas: Visión de su Trayectoria en México.* Mexico City: El Colegio de Mexico, Centro Mexicano para la Filantropía.

Villarreal, Magdalena. 2014. "Regimes of Value in Mexican Household Financial Practices." *Current Anthropology* 55, no. 9: 30–39.

Von Bertrab, Etienne. 2003. "Guadalajara's Water Crisis and the Fate of Lake Chapala: A Reflection of Poor Water Management in Mexico." *Environment and Urbanization* 15, no. 2: 127–140.

Vulliamy, Ed. 2011. "Ciudad Juarez Is All of Our Futures: This Is the Inevitable War of Capitalism Gone Mad." *The Guardian,* June 20, 2011. http://www.theguardian.com/commentisfree/2011/jun/20/war-capitalism-mexico-drug-cartels.

Waldby, Catherine, and Robert Mitchell. 2006. *Tissue Economies: Blood, Organs, and Cell Lines in Late Capitalism.* Durham, N.C.: Duke University Press.

Wallace, Bob, and Roderick Wallace. 2016. "Ebola's Ecologies: Agro-Economics and Epidemiology in West Africa." *New Left Review* 102: 1–13.

Weber, Max. 1946. *Essays in Sociology*. New York, N.Y.: Oxford University Press.

Weiner, Daniel, Michael McClean, James Kaufman, and Daniel Brooks. 2013. "The Central American Epidemic of CKD." *Clinical Journal of the American Society of Nephrology* 8, no. 3: 504–511.

Wesseling, Catharina, Jennifer Crowe, and Christer Hogstedt. 2013. "The Epidemic of Chronic Kidney Disease of Unknown Etiology in Mesoamerica: A Call for Interdisciplinary Research and Action." *American Journal of Public Health* 103, no. 11: 1927–1930.

Wesseling, Catharina, Berna van Wendel de Joode, Jennifer Crowe, Ralf Rittner, Sanati Negin, Christer Hogstedt, and Kristina Jakobsson. 2015. "Mesoamerican Nephropathy: Geographical Distribution and Time Trends of Chronic Kidney Disease Mortality between 1970 and 2012 in Costa Rica." *Occupational & Environmental Medicine* 72, no. 10: 714–721.

White, Susan, Richard Hirth, Beatriz Mahíllo, Beatriz Domínquez-Gil, Francis Delmonico, . . . and Alan Leichtman. 2014. "The Global Diffusion of Organ Transplantation: Trends, Drivers and Policy Implications." *Bulletin of the World Health Organization* 92, no. 11: 826–835.

WHO. 2016. "International Expert Consultation on Chronic Kidney Disease of Unknown Etiology." Report, Colombo, Sri Lanka, April 27–29, 2016. http://www.searo.who.int/srilanka/documents/report_international_expert_consultation_on_ckdu.pdf?ua=1.

Whyte, David. 2015. *How Corrupt Is Britain?* London: Pluto Press.

Whyte, Susan. 2012. "Chronicity and Control: Framing 'Noncommunicable Diseases' in Africa." *Anthropology & Medicine* 19, no. 1: 63–74.

Wild, Sarah, Goika Roglic, Anders Green, Richard Sicree, and Hilary King. 2004. "Global Prevalence of Diabetes: Estimates for the Year 2000 and Projections for 2030." *Diabetes Care* 27, no. 5: 1047–1053.

Wilson, Christopher, and Gerardo Silva. 2013. "Mexico's Latest Poverty Statistics." The Wilson Centre-Mexico Institute. www.wilsoncenter.org/sites/default/files/Poverty_Statistics_Mexico_2013.pdf.

Wittgenstein, Ludvik. 1953. *Philosophical Investigations*. Oxford: Blackwell.

Wolf, Eric. 1982. *Europe and the People without History*. Berkeley: University of California Press.

Wright, Emily. 2016. *Mapping Mesoamerican Nephropathy: Biomedical, Socio-political and Moral Dimensions of a Contested Epidemic*. Academic thesis, Brown University.

INDEX

anthropocene, 149–150. *See also* Tsing, Anna

Antiguo Hospital Civil: dialysis and transplant facilities, 44–45; explanations of, 21, 43–45, 48, 59, 87, 153n12; history of, 8–10; transplant scandal, 23, 114–130

Appadurai, Arjun, 72, 111, 157n2 (chap. 4)

Arendt, Hannah, 36, 63, 112. *See also* labor of sickness

aristolochia, explanation of, 134, 158n1 (chap. 7)

autoconstrucción, 56, 57, 155n1

Auyero, Javier, 11, 117

Balkan nephropathy, 134

bioavailability, 29

biocapital, 95

bioeconomy, 95

biopolitics, 14, 18, 20, 33, 52; arrangements of, 19; conceptual framework, 52, 54, 55, 72; explanation of, 154n15; of indifference, 64, 73; regimes of, 34, 52; specific forms, 14

biopsy: diagnosis of CKD, 4, 16, 46, 80, 88–89, 132; explanation of, 153n8; regarding CKDu, 135

biosocial, 45; biosociality, 102; CKD as, 146

biovalue, 95

Bornstein, Erica, 102

Briggs, Charles, and Clara Mantini-Briggs, 133, 142

bureaucracy, bureaucratization, 101; bureaucratic document, 22, 76, 77, 79; bureaucratic violence, 92; crafted bureaucracy, 157n10; work of, 75, 90–92. *See also* Weber, Max

care: care-giving and gendered aspects, 12, 53, 155n13; concept of, 149

Caritas, 7, 48, 107

Carlos Slim Foundation, 101, 102, 109

CENATRA (centro nacional de trasplantes), 42, 118, 158n2 (chap. 6)

CENCAM (Consortium for the Epidemic of Nephropathy in Central America and Mexico), 139, 158n4 (chap. 7)

CETOT (council of organ and tissue transplant) 118, 122

Chapala lake: emergence of CKDu, 138, 139, 142, 143, 149, 158n5 (chap. 7); living with CKD, 95, 131; location, 4; pollution, 4, 137–139, 159n6; poverty, 140; toxicity, 4, 137–139

charitable associations, 98, 99, 101–103, 105, 109, 110, 112; the work of, 101. *See also* philanthropy

chronic kidney disease (CKD), xiii; definition, 2; diagnostics, 16; etiology, x, 3, 15, 16, 43, 135; material ground of, 35; moral burden of, 3, 4, 131; rise of, 14, 15, 17

chronic kidney disease of unknown origin: Chapala, 4, 131, 132; epidemiology, 16; etiology, x, 15, 17, 43, 132, 133, 134; explanation, 4, 15, 35, 132–140, 143–146, 153n9; global south, 133, 134; Mesoamerican nephropathy, 15, 134; residual unknown, 43; symptoms of, 5; worksite, 133, 140–143. *See also* Mesoamerican nephropathy

Coca-Cola, explanation for CKD, 4

COFEPRIS (Comisión Federal para la Protección contra Riesgos Sanitarios), 105, 127

Cohen, Lawrence, 27, 94; development of organ transplantation, 28

compliance, 102; with dialysis at home, 60, 61; with diet, 3, 5, 7, 82, 83, 85, 87; with medications, 86

Contraloria del Estado de Jalisco (Office of the State Comptroller and General Auditor), 119, 125, 127

creatinine, 80, 83, 87, 88; explanation of, 157n5

Crowley-Matoka, Megan, 27, 38, 40, 41, 90, 91, 94, 102, 155n13

Das, Veena, 54, 129. *See also* everyday violence

diabetes: cause of CKD, x, 15, 16, 42, 132, 135; co-morbidity, 57–59, 71, 138; rise of, x, 4, 14, 23, 154n6. *See also* Montoya, Michael

ABOUT THE AUTHOR

CIARA KIERANS is reader in social anthropology in the Department of Public Health and Policy at the University of Liverpool. Her research focuses on ethnographic studies of medical practice, the biopolitical consequences of medical technologies, and the political economic conditions that ground them. She has conducted ethnographic research in Ireland focusing on embodiment, organ recipiency, and the moral discourses of gift-giving; in the UK on organ donation, institutional practice, and the production of race and genetic identities, and in Mexico on chronic kidney disease and transplant medicine with a focus on the role of the welfare state and market in producing catastrophic poverty and social suffering. She has written widely for both anthropological and interdisciplinary audiences.

Printed in the United States
By Bookmasters